Arthritis

Professor John Marcus Thompson

Emeritus Professor, Faculty of Medicine,
University of Western Ontario
Former Chief of Rheumatology,
St Joseph's Medical Centre, London, Canada

Class Publishing • London

First edition published in Canada by Key Porter Books Limited,
Toronto, Canada 1995
Reprinted 2000
Reprinted 2003
First UK edition 2004

The authors and publishers welcome feedback from the users of this book.
Please contact the publishers.

Class Publishing (London) Ltd
Barb House, Barb Mews, London W6 7PA, UK
Telephone: 020 7371 2119
Fax: 020 7371 2878 [International +4420]
Email: post@class.co.uk

A CIP catalogue record for this book is available from the British Library.

ISBN 1 85959 106 X

Edited by Gillian Clarke
Designed and typeset by Martin Bristow
Illustrations by Martyn Lengden
Indexed by Val Elliston

Printed and bound in Finland by WS Bookwell, Juva

Contents

Foreword

A common aphorism states that knowledge is power. This principle certainly applies to consumers of medical care. Recent changes in health-care delivery require people to make more of their own decisions about how and where they will obtain care. Research findings clearly show that people who understand their illness and actively participate in treatment decisions have better outcomes and greater satisfaction.

The new emphasis on health-care costs and efficiency means that doctors often don't have adequate time to talk with their patients. Studies have consistently shown that the doctor's office is not a good setting for learning. Also, patients are often too upset, or too deferential to the doctor, to press for answers. Moreover, the doctor can't judge exactly what each patient needs to learn. Given these realities, patients must increasingly take responsibility for educating themselves.

This eminently readable book is a comprehensive resource for people with arthritis who wish to learn more about this very common group of illnesses. They should use it to make themselves more informed participants in the care of their illness, and to identify specific issues to discuss with their physicians. Most important, they should use it to help themselves feel more in charge of the illness, and of their lives.

Robert F. Meenan, MD, MPH, MBA
Director, Boston University School
of Public Health

Author's Note

I've gone into detail in many sections of this book because I believe patients want and need detail. I feel strongly that in order to have the best possible outcome and avoid misadventure, patients must know as much about their arthritis as their doctor knows. This book is not simply an introduction; it is a manual, to be referred to repeatedly as circumstances change.

But because things do change – in particular with drug dosages and precautions – specifics should be checked with a health professional (a physician, pharmacist or nurse) if there is a discrepancy between what I have written and what the reader has been told.

Acknowledgements

The professionals of the London, Ontario, office of the Arthritis Society, and in particular Nancy Ambrogio, Janet Goodhoofd, Joanne Cuttiford and Tammy Regier, have contributed significantly to this book, both as constructive critics and (in the section on therapy) as co-authors. They deserve my public thanks.

Several patients read individual sections and helped me with their comments. Of course, in a larger sense, my patients have made an enormous contribution over the years to my understanding of arthritis. My thanks, though, go beyond that. Few non-physicians can guess the rewards arising from what is rather cryptically called 'the doctor–patient relationship'. For trust, for understanding, for friendship, for all these I thank those I've been permitted to know and care for over the last quarter century.

Finally, in countless ways Ana Thompson made this book possible.

Thank you all.

John M. Thompson, MD

Dedication

When I first met Carol, she was 24 years old. Her joint symptoms had begun four years earlier with the birth of her son, improved when she got pregnant again and returned for good when her daughter was born just a few months before that first visit.

Carol died 19 years later, almost to the day.

Over those years I got to know Carol well. We went through so much together: countless surgical procedures; virtually every drug then available; complications of arthritis that I had never seen before and have seldom seen since. Carol was in and out of hospital innumerable times, particularly in her final years. A crisis would force her to come in, and as soon as she was even partially better she would press to be discharged, to be home with her family. Finally, her life became impossible. She anticipated her death, and both she and Paul, her husband, were ready for it.

Carol had a mischievous, infectious sense of humour. She wasn't above taking gentle pokes at 'the doctor', and I took these as a compliment. She shared a birthday with my wife, and every May 8 a card and a box of homemade cookies would be delivered to my office. The last few years, it was Paul or one of her children, now grown, who came by.

Carol dealt with her disease with grace and acceptance. Probably more than any other patient, she taught me about arthritis, about being a doctor, about living. This book is for her.

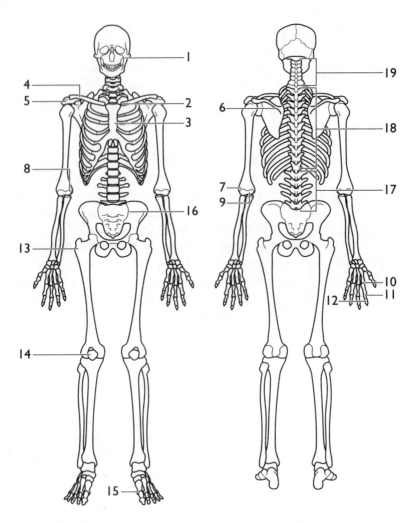

1 temporomandibular (TM or jaw) joint
2 sternoclavicular joint
3 sternum (breast bone)
4 clavicle (collar bone)
5 acromioclavicular joint
6 scapula (shoulder blade)
7 lateral epicondyle

8 medial epicondyle
9 elbow
10 metacarpophalangeal (MCP) joint
11 proximal interphalangeal (PIP) joint
12 distal interphalangeal (DIP) joint

13 greater trochanter
14 patella (knee cap)
15 metatarsophalangeal (MTP) joint
16 sacroiliac joint
17 lumbar spine
18 dorsal (thoracic) spine
19 cervical spine

Anatomy of the skeleton

1
First things first

'Rheumatology' is the name given to the medical speciality that deals with people who have problems with their joints. Diagnosis and non-surgical treatment of these is the focus. Because a joint problem is often not the only one the patient has, the speciality spills over to include diseases that also affect muscles, the nerves, the blood, the skin, the kidneys – in fact, almost every part of the body.

I am a rheumatologist. After medical school I went on to spend three years learning the art of general internal medicine, and a further two years working exclusively with people with arthritis. For a little over 30 years I have been a practising rheumatologist. Several days each week, I see patients who are referred to me because of joint pain.

Very often, after I've completed my examination, my patient will ask, 'Tell me, doctor, is it arthritis?' The diagnosis may be one of a dozen very different conditions – osteoarthritis of the big toe, rheumatoid arthritis, back pain and gout are all common – but my answer to that particular question has to be 'Yes'. I then have to go on to explain, because I know that my patient is thinking, 'Wheelchair'.

I explain that 'arthritis' means, literally, 'joint inflammation'. I add that we, doctors and patients, have come to lump just about anything that hurts in the muscles and the skeleton under this heading. My grandparents would have used the term 'rheumatism'.

'Arthritis' includes dozens of different conditions. Some are temporary, some are permanent. Some are harmless and some are disabling. Some are curable, some are not. So the word 'arthritis', as most of us use it, is meaningless. We must be specific. That's the purpose of this book – to be specific, and to give meaning to the specific.

Another term to describe what we often call 'arthritis' or

'rheumatism' is 'musculoskeletal disorder' (MSD). MSDs include joint disease (about 60 per cent), back and neck pain (about 30 per cent) and a wide variety of other problems, including tendinitis and bursitis (about 10 per cent).

Surveys carried out in Britain, Canada and the USA are remarkably consistent. Every year, 15 per cent of the population consult their general practitioner because of an MSD.

Estimates of some of the more common types of adult MSDs are:

- osteoarthritis   1 in 10
- fibromyalgia   4 in 100
- rheumatoid arthritis   1 in 100
- crystal arthritis   1 in 100
- ankylosing spondylitis   1 in 1,000
- psoriatic arthritis   1 in 1,000
- systemic lupus erythematosus   1 in 3,500

How to use this book

This book covers a lot of territory. Chapters 2, 3, 4 and 5 deal with specific types of arthritis, and for most readers just one or two will be of uppermost concern.

There are sections, however, that are generally relevant. The next section, 'How a diagnosis is made', is a good starting point for anyone, particularly someone who has just recently begun to hurt. The distinction between 'inflammatory' and 'non-inflammatory' pain is important.

Chapter 6, 'What's going on?', provides information on symptoms as they crop up in various parts of the body. Some may be part of a larger arthritic problem but many are not. Some aren't important at all, except as a source of worry. This is a 'how-to-do-it' chapter.

Finally, Chapter 7, 'The treatment of arthritis', is very important and generally applicable. Almost every person with pain is treated with pills. Because these may harm as well as help, patients have to learn to recognise side effects as they arise. This chapter should help with that. It also touches on a number of treatment possibilities that may not have been considered.

Obviously, this book is not meant to be read at a single sitting, but to be consulted, and reconsulted, over time.

How a diagnosis is made

Ask any medical student how a diagnosis is made, and she or he will answer, 'Through a complete history, a thorough physical examination and appropriate laboratory tests.'

This response, embedded in the medical profession's collective memory, was recently tested. Researchers in Texas presented a series of arthritis 'cases' to a number of doctors. The problem cases were typical of those seen in practice – osteoarthritis, rheumatoid arthritis, back pain, gout, tendinitis and fibromyalgia were some of them. The doctors were all involved in general internal medicine, some were training to become specialists, and others were their teachers. This was a 'paper' exercise; they didn't see the patients but details of the history and physical examination were provided. They were asked to diagnose each case. To help them, they could order any test they felt was needed. Their performances were compared with the performances of a group of rheumatologists.

The outcome of the exercise was predictable. The doctors-in-training didn't do as well as their teachers, who in turn didn't do as well as the rheumatologists. Experience did count for something. Doctors who had been specialists for at least six years got 80 per cent of the correct answers (the others were around 70 per cent). It also helped if doctors had received some exposure to patients with arthritis. Even two weeks made a big difference.

One fascinating part of the study has particular relevance in today's cost-conscious world: to reach their incorrect diagnoses (three out of ten), the non-rheumatologists far outspent the arthritis doctors on unnecessary tests.

A fourth part should be added: 'and a doctor with relevant experience'. In other words, the cheapest and best 'test' is a referral to an appropriate specialist. This is particularly important in rheumatology because – despite the fact that 'rheumatism' makes up the largest part of general practice – most of today's medical graduates have little or no experience with arthritis.

From the first moment I meet a new patient, I begin to collect information that will help answer two very important questions: 'Is the problem inflammatory or non-inflammatory?' and 'Is the problem local or widespread?'

Inflammatory or non-inflammatory?

The answer to this question is very important. Generally, inflammatory arthritis:

- affects more joints,
- causes more damage and disability,
- is linked more often to problems elsewhere in the body,
- is more likely to be influenced by treatment.

Inflammation, whether due to sunburn, a mosquito bite or inflammatory arthritis, has four features: pain, swelling, redness and warmth. Rheumatoid arthritis, systemic lupus erythematosus (SLE) and gout are quite different but they all share these four characteristics.

Non-inflammatory arthritis (osteoarthritis is by far the most common type) may be painful, reflecting joint damage, and swelling is common. However, redness and warmth are absent unless something else, such as infection or bleeding, is also present. And non-inflammatory forms of arthritis are seldom linked to problems elsewhere in the body.

Widespread or local?

'Widespread' has two meanings. The doctor needs to know not only how many and which joints are affected but also if there is a problem somewhere else in the body that is connected to the joint symptoms.

The greater the number of joints involved, the more likely the problem is to be inflammatory. Symptoms suggesting difficulty in one of the other body systems – the muscles, the skin, the eye, nerves, the lungs, heart and kidney – may indicate one of the 'systemic rheumatic diseases' – inflammatory conditions such as rheumatoid arthritis and SLE.

'Local' means that the problem is confined to joints or nearby tissues. Most non-inflammatory forms of arthritis, and occasionally some inflammatory ones as well, are local, and usually involve only a few joints.

What is the pattern of pain and stiffness?

How the patient feels at certain times of the day, and for how long, can provide important clues towards a diagnosis. Here are some of the questions doctors ask:

- *How long does it take for you to get loosened up in the morning?*
  'Morning stiffness' refers to the pain and difficulty with movement that patients with inflammation feel upon awakening. It isn't just in the involved joints – it's felt all over. It's in the muscles and in the joints.

  Morning stiffness makes it difficult, even temporarily impossible, to bathe or get dressed. The more activity the person manages, the sooner the problem gets better, but it may take hours to do so. In people with a major flare-up of arthritis, morning stiffness may even continue all day. Its duration is a pretty good measure of how active the arthritis is.

  Stiffening up – the medical term is 'gelling' – after sitting quietly later in the day is a similar symptom. Fortunately, gelling is considerably briefer than morning stiffness.

  Non-inflammatory arthritis also has some morning stiffness, but it gets better quickly with activity, usually within a few minutes.

  In contrast to inflammatory stiffness, which improves with activity, non-inflammatory joint pain gets worse the more the joint is used. People with osteoarthritis of the hip, for example, are at their worst at the end of the day.

- *How is your energy level?*
  Fatigue almost always accompanies inflammatory arthritis. People often find it harder to deal with than pain or stiffness. Among the non-inflammatory forms of arthritis, only fibromyalgia causes fatigue of similar degree.

- *Do you have pain at night?*
  The pain of inflammatory arthritis is often bad at night.
  This is particularly true if the spine and the shoulders are
  involved. People may get to sleep without difficulty, only to
  wake in pain in the small hours of the morning. In contrast,
  people with non-inflammatory pain generally feel better
  with rest.

- *How did it all start, and how has it behaved since then?*
  The more sudden the onset of the problem, the more likely
  it is to be inflammatory. Gout and polymyalgia rheumatica
  typically 'explode' overnight. Osteoarthritis, however, may
  be hardly noticeable at the start. People often have
  difficulty remembering when it first began.
     Non-inflammatory progression tends to be slow and
  steady over the years. Symptoms that disappear completely,
  only to flare up again later, are indicators of inflammation.

- *Have any joints been warm, red or swollen?*
  In clear-cut joint inflammation, there is redness and local
  heat in addition to pain and swelling. However, the
  spectrum ranges from the extreme inflammation of an
  attack of gout to, in some cases, a minor puffiness of
  knuckles in rheumatoid arthritis. In fact, the entire range of
  inflammatory signs may be seen at different times in the
  same person.
     In non-inflammatory arthritis, joint swelling frequently
  occurs but clues to inflammation, such as warmth and
  redness, are absent. There are exceptions. As already
  mentioned, infection or bleeding due to injury may mimic
  inflammation. In nodal osteoarthritis, a common variant,
  warmth and redness may fool the unwary.

- *What's been the response to treatment?*
  As a rule, most of the non-steroidal anti-inflammatory
  drugs (NSAIDs), such as ibuprofen, naproxen and aspirin,
  are only modestly effective in most forms of arthritis.
  However, there are exceptions, and if a patient describes
  spectacular improvement in symptoms with treatment, it
  can help with the diagnosis. For example, patients with

inflammatory back pain due to ankylosing spondylitis, when started on a regular and adequate dose of an NSAID, will suddenly be able to sleep through the night. Similarly, the spectacular inflammation of a gouty toe can be wiped out if the right NSAID is started at the right time.

Once it is known whether the problem is inflammatory or not, the next task is to see if the history will lead to a more specific diagnosis. Doctors rely a great deal on what the patient can tell them about the pattern of the arthritis, any symptoms in addition to joint pain, the family history and the medication history.

The pattern of the arthritis

'Pattern' refers not only to the location in the body but also to the behaviour of the arthritis. Is just one joint – or are only a few – the problem? Is the problem mostly in large joints? Is the problem symmetrical – that is, does it involve similar joints on both right and left sides? Are the hand joints involved, and, if so, which ones? Does the arthritis come and go, or is it gradually getting worse? Most patterns are not unique to a specific disease, but recognising a pattern helps to narrow the possibilities. A few, in fact, are unique, making the diagnosis easy.

Common patterns include:

- Acute monoarthritis – a single joint is suddenly very painful. If this has happened before and the patient is an adult man, the chances are that this is due to gout or chondrocalcinosis. If this is a first attack, however, infection or bleeding into the joint have to be considered.

- Chronic polyarthritis – persistent involvement of many joints. If just one or two joints are involved, and they are large ones such as the knee and the hip, osteoarthritis is a strong bet. If many joints are involved (especially small ones) and both hands are affected, rheumatoid arthritis and nodal osteoarthritis are the most likely diagnoses.

- Spinal pain – both inflammatory (spondylitis) and non-inflammatory (osteoarthritis) problems may cause low back pain, but night pain helps distinguish one from the other.

- Pain felt in muscles – particularly the muscles of the upper arms and the thighs and buttocks – isn't usually caused by muscle inflammation. The problem is more likely to be nearby arthritis, bursitis or tendinitis.

Symptoms in addition to joint pain

In many types of arthritis, inflammation is not confined to joints. As mentioned earlier, other parts of the body may be affected. The rheumatologist then looks for evidence of 'systemic disease' – inflammation of other body systems.

Clues to this may be non-specific. Profound fatigue, appetite and weight loss, fever or night sweats are very important symptoms. Or clues may be very specific, and quite helpful in pinpointing the rheumatic syndrome. For example, pleurisy (knife-like chest pain on breathing deeply) may be part of systemic lupus erythematosus, whilst a man with Reiter's syndrome may report pain on urination and a discharge from his penis.

There isn't an organ system that isn't involved in at least one kind of arthritis – the skin (and hair and nails), the eyes, nose and mouth, the lungs, the heart, the gut, the kidneys and the nervous system. Organ system involvement is not only important for making a diagnosis. It also has important implications for treatment and for the long-term outlook.

Family history of arthritis

Knowledge that other family members have had arthritis is usually not terribly helpful. Joint problems are very common, and people seldom know the exact diagnosis of a parent or a cousin. However, some types of arthritis do have a definite tendency to occur in families, and this information can be useful. The best-known example is ankylosing spondylitis. Gout and rheumatoid arthritis also tend to run in families.

Other drugs taken

A list of all medication taken, including over-the-counter products (no prescription needed), is important. Occasionally, drugs as different as procainamide (for heart irregularities), minocycline (for acne) or diuretics (for high blood pressure) will cause serious arthritis problems.

Examining for arthritis

Many patients are surprised when I ask them to put on a hospital gown. They obviously expect a quick look at the painful area and a diagnosis. I do make 'snap' diagnoses, but there is always a risk: arthritis may be the tip of the iceberg, a sign of a condition that affects other parts of the body. If it is, the organ systems involved may provide the clue to the correct diagnosis. A complete physical examination should be the rule.

The general examination

This examination is particularly important in determining or confirming if there are systemic aspects to the problem.

I ask the patient to strip down to underclothes and slip on a gown. Undressing is important because, in addition to checking blood pressure and testing reflexes, I'm going to be examining the chest, heart and abdomen. In a woman, a breast examination may be necessary. When I do this I try to explain why it's necessary, but sometimes I forget. Here, or in any other part of the examination, the patient should feel free to ask the reasons for the procedure and to request that a friend or partner be present.

The musculoskeletal examination

Like the general physical examination, this is tailored to the problem being considered. Someone who has severe low back pain will be examined differently from someone with a painful knee. Nevertheless, a quick survey of the skeleton, taking less than two or three minutes, can give a good idea of what's normal and what's not.

If this quick 'screening' picks up a problem, the suspicious area can be assessed more thoroughly.

The physician's sense of feel is important. Touch can detect problems of joint warmth, swelling, crepitus (grinding) or resistance.

Joint warmth points to inflammation. Usually it refers to a joint being warmer than the area around it, but some joints, the knee especially, are normally cooler than the surrounding tissues. Use the back of your hand to feel the temperature of your kneecap and compare that with your thigh and shin. If the three areas are equally warm, you've got an inflammatory problem with your knee.

Joint swelling may or may not be caused by inflammation. Swelling may reflect fluid within the joint, thickened tissues around the joint, or bony overgrowth around the edges of the joint. If fluid is discovered in the joint, it can be extracted and tested (see 'Laboratory tests', below).

Joint crepitus is the term for the grinding sensation that is felt, and sometimes heard, when the joint is being moved. It always means that there's a problem with the tissues of the joint. A good examiner can tell the difference between the crepitus caused by roughened cartilage (the 'gristle' at the bone ends), by inflamed synovial tissue (the membrane that lines the joint), or by bone rubbing on bone when the overlying cartilage has been worn away.

Joint resistance, when the physician attempts to move the joint through a full range of movement, may be the first clue to a problem in that joint. This is particularly true in the case of the shoulder, the hip and the back, where pain may be felt some distance from its true source. A good example is hip pain: it's supposed to be felt in the groin, but some patients deny pain there and complain bitterly of pain in the front of the thigh, or even in the knee. The knee looks normal, but, when the doctor tries to bring the hip up to a right angle and rotate it inwards, it just won't go – and the patient repeats that the knee is hurting.

The joints that are involved (as determined by examination) may fit a pattern. This is particularly so in the hands (see box).

- Pattern 1 – a number of DIP joints alone, or in combination with PIP joints, almost always point to nodal osteoarthritis.

- Pattern 2 – a number of MCP joints alone, or more commonly combined with PIP joints, almost always point to rheumatoid arthritis.

Hand patterns

The end knuckle of a finger is called the DIP (distal inter-phalangeal) joint.

The middle knuckle is the PIP (proximal interphalangeal) joint.

The knuckle at the base of the finger is the MCP (metacarpo-phalangeal) joint.

Laboratory tests

The list of tests used in the initial evaluation of the problem is surprisingly short. The laboratory is being used to address the basic questions: 'inflammatory or not?', 'systemic or not?'

Later, particularly if a systemic form of arthritis has been diagnosed on the 'first pass', more tests may be needed. But if the history and physical examination suggest neither an inflammatory nor a systemic problem, the only reason for further testing is to help to guide treatment.

The following tests are commonly done. The complete blood count (CBC), erythrocyte sedimentation rate (ESR) or C-reactive protein (CRP) and kidney tests are performed most often, to help with diagnosis or to guide treatment. Rheumatoid factor (RF), antinuclear antibody (ANA), joint aspiration and X-rays are done to answer specific questions about diagnosis.

It is important to know that tests can mislead. It's common for a blood test to give a 'positive' result for gout, SLE or even rheumatoid arthritis in someone who doesn't have any of these diseases.

Complete blood count (CBC)

The complete blood count involves counting the number of red blood cells, white blood cells and platelets – the formed elements of the blood. Some kinds of arthritis, and some kinds of treatment, can affect any or all of the three types.

Because red blood cells carry oxygen from the lungs to the body, white blood cells are one of the body's main means of dealing with infection, and platelets are very important in blood clotting, problems with any one of them may cause real trouble.

- Anaemia (a low red blood cell count) is common in inflammatory arthritis. Usually this reflects the fact that the bone marrow, which is where blood cells are made, just isn't able to keep up production when inflammation is present, even if it has all the ingredients, including enough iron. But anaemia can also be due to arthritis medicine, particularly NSAIDs such as aspirin, which may cause bleeding from a stomach or duodenal ulcer, and a resulting low red blood cell count.

- Low white blood cell counts and low numbers of platelets may occur, separately or together, in some kinds of arthritis. Unfortunately, similar problems may be caused by some of the drugs used to treat arthritis, so the situation can be confusing.

Sedimentation rate and CRP

The 'sedimentation rate' is an old test but it still has a useful place in medicine. Blood is normally a suspension of cells – red blood cells, mostly. If blood is left to stand in a test-tube, it will separate out – the red blood cells at the bottom, the clear yellow plasma at the top. The speed at which red blood cells settle out (sediment) varies depending on a number of circumstances. Inflammation is one of them. A normal sedimentation rate is 20 millimetres per hour or less; in some forms of arthritis it may be as high as 80 millimetres per hour.

A high sedimentation rate can confirm suspicions of inflammation – but, like many other tests, the results may be high (elevated) in conditions other than arthritis, and even in 'normal' people. Nor is the test a good way to follow the course of the disease. To answer the question 'Is the patient getting better or worse?' a few questions and a quick examination are far better.

The CRP (C-reactive protein) is a blood test that is starting to be used to replace the sedimentation rate. It can be automated, so it's cheaper to perform, and it's less likely to be fooled by non-inflammatory conditions than is the sedimentation rate. It is also a good test for measuring treatment effect and response.

Kidney tests – blood creatinine and BUN, and urinalysis

Kidney problems are usually not evident from the patient's history and physical examination but are important because they may be a major complication of some kinds of arthritis. In systemic lupus erythematosus, kidney inflammation may lead to kidney failure. An abnormal urinalysis may point the way not only to the correct diagnosis but also to the correct treatment.

Creatinine and blood urea nitrogen (BUN) are chemical substances excreted by the kidney. In the presence of reduced kidney function, which usually happens without the patient being aware of it, the levels of these chemicals in the blood rise.

Impaired kidney function, not necessarily due to arthritis, is common in older people and in those taking certain medication. Many of the drugs used for arthritis affect the kidneys and, although this isn't usually important, in someone who already has a problem it could be critical. It's vital that treatment not cause already badly functioning kidneys to become worse. To detect patients at risk, these tests are valuable.

Rheumatoid factor (RF)

This blood test, which detects a protein present in many people with rheumatoid arthritis, is unfortunately neither 100 per cent sensitive for everyone with rheumatoid arthritis, nor specific for it.

In early rheumatoid arthritis, RF will not be detected in at least a third (some think the figure is closer to half) of patients. It is also occasionally found in other forms of arthritis and in some other chronic (long-term) diseases. Nevertheless, if RF is found in someone whose story and examination are consistent with rheumatoid arthritis, the diagnosis is basically confirmed.

This test should not be done on anyone with general aches and pains. It should be limited to those who have physical findings consistent with rheumatoid arthritis. This way, the test is not only diagnostic but also tells the doctor something about that person's future (see 'Rheumatoid arthritis' in Chapter 2).

Antinuclear antibody (ANA)

The ANA is a blood test used in the diagnosis of systemic lupus erythematosus (SLE). As mentioned above, in rheumatoid arthritis the RF test is negative in a large number of patients in the early stages. But in patients with SLE a negative ANA test is very rare, occurring in 5 per cent or less. So a negative ANA reassures the doctor (with about 95 per cent certainty) that his or her patient doesn't have that disease. A positive test is not as helpful, because it turns up in many 'normal' people, and can be found in quite a number of other diseases as well. In fact, because SLE is relatively rare, it is far more likely that a positive ANA will be a 'false' positive rather than a 'true' positive.

A positive ANA is just the first step. There must be other proof, from the patient's history, or examination, or from the lab, before SLE can be diagnosed.

Joint aspiration

This is one test that often turns up the 'crucial piece' in the puzzle.

Drawing a specimen of fluid from a swollen joint, using a needle and syringe, and sending it to the laboratory can supply a great deal of information. Analysis of the white blood cell count helps make the distinction between inflammatory and non-inflammatory arthritis. The fluid can also be tested for infection, and examination using a microscope will reveal the crystals of gout and chondrocalcinosis if they are present.

Unless the doctor is absolutely certain of the cause, fluid from a swollen joint should always be obtained and examined. This is not as horrible as it sounds: only a small amount of fluid is needed, and this can usually be obtained using a very fine needle. When this is done by an experienced doctor, the discomfort is no more than is felt when a blood sample is taken from the arm.

X-rays and other images

In the routine assessment of arthritis, X-rays should be used even less than laboratory tests. They hardly ever help make the diagnosis in people with recent-onset arthritis. Still, they may confirm suspicions of certain specific problems, such as:

- fractures,

- infections involving bone,

- cancer involving bone,

- chondrocalcinosis, a form of arthritis that involves calcium deposits.

They are also used to determine the extent of joint damage, particularly if joint surgery is being considered.

Other ways to look at bone, joints and soft tissues include:

- ultrasound,

- bone scans (nuclear isotope scanning),

- magnetic resonance imaging (MRI),

- computed tomography (CT scans).

These forms of imaging should be used even less frequently than X-rays. However, they can sometimes provide the critical piece in the puzzle, if done with specific questions in mind.

2
Inflammatory arthritis

'No-name' inflammatory arthritis

Arthritis is a problem for Kevin, and Kevin is a problem for me. Kevin is a 28-year-old cook. It's clear his problem is inflammatory. For three months now he has had joint pain with typical inflammatory features: swelling, slight warmth, significant and prolonged stiffness first thing in the morning. He has responded fairly well to an NSAID. So far the problem is most obviously in his right knee and both wrists. His fingers are stiff, too, but there is no obvious swelling or restricted movement in them.

He has absolutely no other symptoms or physical findings that might help me 'pigeon-hole' him. His blood tests have shown a slight anaemia, a sedimentation rate test result that is mildly elevated and a negative rheumatoid factor. I know that if I X-ray his painful joints I'll simply be wasting money.

I've recommended a trial of hydroxychloroquine, an additional drug that often helps in a broad range of inflammatory arthritides (that's the plural for 'arthritis'). Kevin is willing to try it, but first he'd like me to answer two simple questions – 'What have I got?' and 'What's going to happen to me?'

Rheumatologists see a lot of people like Kevin. In fact, just about half of all patients with an inflammatory problem involving multiple joints are initially undiagnosable, despite the doctors' best efforts.

Recent studies have attempted to look at this issue in more detail. Their conclusions are going to help me give Kevin some sort of answer.

First, Kevin is unlikely to have rheumatoid arthritis (RA). We knew that women are roughly three times more likely to get RA, but we now know that for people under 45 the ratio is 6 to 1. Over all, a man's risk of developing RA is estimated at 14 in

100,000 each year, but under 45 the risk is only 2 in 100,000. So, with a negative RF test, RA is very unlikely for Kevin.

In a large American study, patients who, like Kevin, couldn't be given a definite diagnosis at their first visit were followed up for several years. In just over half, the problem cleared up completely without a diagnosis ever being made. This is in sharp contrast to those who had clear-cut RA on their first visit. Of those, barely 7 per cent were in remission after three years.

Those who didn't clear up were about equally divided into three groups: some developed clear-cut RA, some continued to mystify, and some either went on to more uncommon forms of arthritis (such as SLE) or were felt, in retrospect, never to have had inflammatory arthritis.

The chance of the problem clearing up and going away lessens as time goes by. Kevin has had symptoms for only three months, so he has an almost 60 per cent chance of remission. If he had been in trouble for over 18 months, that chance would be only 15 per cent.

So Kevin has a lot going for him. He's under 45, his symptoms are recent, his RF test is negative and his rheumatologist can't pin a label on him. This is one time when no diagnosis is a good diagnosis.

Rheumatoid arthritis (RA)

Sandra is a slender 35-year-old woman who walks with the grace of a professional dancer, which she is. She is also a delight. Her bubbling optimism is infectious and I look forward to her visits.

She first came to me a year ago, when her family physician asked me to see her as soon as possible. She'd been unwell for three months. The slightest effort exhausted her. A month earlier, her knees had become painful and swollen. The PIP and MCP joints (see Figure 2.1 on page 23) of her hands had followed, then her elbows and ankles. To get out of bed and into the shower each morning was extremely difficult. Her whole body was sore and stiff, and only started to improve at mid-morning. Movement and a hot shower seemed to speed the loosening-up process but later in the day, when she rested and then resumed movement, she re-experienced this stiffness, if only for a few minutes.

Her family doctor had asked her to take eight to twelve aspirin a day. He had prescribed the 'enteric-coated' variety (the coating protects the stomach from the aspirin). These had helped take the edge off her pain but had not really affected the swelling.

The laboratory test results her doctor sent along included:

- a red blood cell count showing mild anaemia,

- a normal sedimentation rate,

- a negative antinuclear antibody (ANA) test,

- a negative rheumatoid factor test,

- a normal urinalysis,

- normal X-rays of hands and feet.

Sandra's general physical examination was normal as well. I paid particular attention to her heart and lungs but heard nothing suspicious. I felt for rheumatoid nodules just below the elbow but found none.

However, the second and third MCP joints of both hands were swollen, as were several PIP joints. I could feel the tension behind the swelling as I pressed firmly with my fingertips; it hurt her, and she told me so. Her wrists and elbows also hurt when I tried to make them bend and extend fully. She hadn't mentioned her feet but I wasn't surprised when she pulled away as I squeezed the width of her foot at the MTP joints.

At this point, I was reasonably certain that the diagnosis was rheumatoid arthritis (RA). But polyarthritis – arthritis involving many joints – that is symmetrical, particularly in a young woman, can result from other causes such as the following.

• Systemic lupus erythematosus

This is the possibility that seems to worry most patients. Young women are commonly the target, and the arthritis in the early stages of SLE may be identical. The fact that Sandra had no symptoms except joint pain and fatigue and had a normal urinalysis was encouraging. The negative ANA test was even more helpful; a negative result is rare in someone with SLE.

- **Psoriasis**

There was no evidence of psoriasis in the usual places – behind Sandra's ears, at the back of her scalp, over her elbows.

- **Inflammatory bowel disease**

Similarly, there was no hint of bowel symptoms that might suggest Crohn's disease or ulcerative colitis.

The only thing that made me hesitate to diagnose RA was the fact that Sandra's joint symptoms had been present for only a month. Other kinds of joint inflammation can be mistaken for RA – such as the arthritis sometimes seen in measles, hepatitis or parvovirus B19 infection. (Parvovirus is a very common childhood infection. Sometimes an adult who wasn't infected as a child catches it and develops an arthritis that looks a lot like RA but usually clears up in weeks.) We really needed to wait a few weeks to see if things would improve.

I gave Sandra a prescription for naproxen, an alternative to aspirin, and gave her a follow-up appointment in two weeks. On her return, she felt considerably better. The pain had improved, she was sleeping better and her fatigue was somewhat less. But her swollen joints remained. I arranged for a physiotherapist from the Arthritis Society to see her. I also suggested adding an additional drug to the naproxen, but Sandra wasn't keen on the idea so I didn't press the point.

Two months later, Sandra reported a three-week period when she had no symptoms. Unfortunately, this was followed by a return of all the symptoms, now worse than ever. She was stiff almost until noon each day, and by mid-afternoon she had to lie down and rest because of fatigue. Her joints remained swollen.

It was now clear that more than naproxen was needed, so I added hydroxychloroquine. That was nine months ago. At present, Sandra is experiencing only a few minutes of morning stiffness but still tires easily. She has a few tender knuckles but the swelling is gone.

True to her basically optimistic self, Sandra is delighted with her present condition, and has started to press me about when she can stop the medication. I'm a bit more pessimistic. Although her RA is no threat to her as long as it stays at this level, I know from past experience that this may not last.

Rheumatoid arthritis is the most common type of chronic inflammatory arthritis. It can affect any joint, large or small.

A dozen or more joints may be affected at any one time. Other parts of the body may be involved in the inflammatory process. Its cause is not known but it is considered to be an autoimmune disease: the immune system, designed to help the body fight off infection, is somehow triggered to react against a person's own tissues. White blood cells – in particular T lymphocytes – are right in the centre of this immune attack. (Doctors have noted that if patients with rheumatoid arthritis are infected with HIV, a retrovirus that causes the T-cell count to drop, their arthritis improves.)

Who gets rheumatoid arthritis?

Rheumatoid arthritis affects at least one out of every 100 North American and European whites. The figure is much lower for Japanese and Chinese and for African blacks, but is the same for North American blacks. In some North American native populations, such as the Chippewa of Minnesota and the Pima of Arizona, it is even higher – about one in 20.

Most women develop RA in their 30s and 40s, most men a few decades later, but in both it can also develop in old age. By age 65 almost 5 per cent of women and 2 per cent of men will have RA. Roughly three women have RA for every man but the sex difference tends to narrow with increasing age. For some reason, the prevalence of RA in women (but not in men) has gone down over the last 20 years.

Rheumatoid arthritis has a slight tendency to run in families – blood relatives of someone with RA have a risk of about 3 per cent instead of the general risk of 1 per cent. If one twin has RA, the risk to the other twin is from around 5–7 per cent (for non-identical twins) to 30 per cent (for identical twins).

Although studies of race and family point to the influence of genetic factors, environmental factors must also play a part. In South Africa, for example, one black group has RA much less often than the white population, but only in a rural setting. When these people move to the city, they acquire RA at the same rate as whites.

Criteria for RA*

If one or more of the following is present, the problem may be rheumatoid arthritis. Referral to a rheumatologist – soon – is recommended.

- Morning stiffness of 30 minutes or more

- Three or more swollen joints

- Tenderness in the MCP or MTP joints when squeezed from the side

* Compiled from an article by Professor Paul Emery, University of Leeds, published in 2002.

How is rheumatoid arthritis diagnosed?

We don't know the cause of RA, so we can't identify it by testing for the cause. Instead, we rely on a group of features, or criteria, that fit most people who are considered to have RA and exclude, as far as possible, those with other kinds of arthritis.

These criteria aren't infallible. There is still a chance that someone who meets the criteria will eventually prove to have something else. But that rarely happens, and treatment tends to be similar in such cases anyway.

Morning stiffness
Morning stiffness isn't unique to RA. It's seen in many kinds of inflammatory arthritis, and in some (such as fibromyalgia) that aren't inflammatory.

This symptom has never been well explained. It has been suggested that the stiffness is due to fluid accumulating in the tissues around joints when the joints are rested, as they are overnight. The duration of morning stiffness is a rough guide to how active RA is at any given moment. In very active RA, it may take until noon to loosen up, and a few people insist it never does. In people who have shown major improvement, morning stiffness may be as brief as five or ten minutes.

Joints affected

What makes RA different from other types of arthritis is that there are so many affected joints, both large and small, both weight-bearing and non-weight-bearing.

The MCP and PIP joints of the hands are almost always affected. The MCP joints of the index and long fingers are particularly vulnerable. Other kinds of arthritis occasionally affect these two joints, but 95 per cent of the time the problem is due to RA.

The MTP joints of the feet are just as commonly inflamed.

Any joint can be affected by RA, however, and in very active disease dozens frequently are. Figure 2.1 gives an idea of how many joints are involved in RA, and how often. The pattern is usually (though not always) similar on both sides of the body. If one elbow, shoulder or wrist is causing grief, the other usually follows.

Rheumatoid nodules

These are bumps – from the size of a kernel of corn to that of a small cherry – that develop under the skin. The most typical location is on the forearm, just below the elbow. Pressure seems to trigger their development; habitually resting a forearm on the arm of a chair or on a table is thought to be a factor. Less commonly, people develop nodules over the Achilles tendon (where the back of a high shoe or boot presses), or over the knuckles of fingers or toes where pressure is applied again and again.

Nodules may be single or in clusters. Some can be moved about under the skin, whereas others seem stuck to the underlying bone. They aren't painful unless they are injured or infected. They may be mistaken for other kinds of bumps, including tophi (deposits of uric acid), seen in some people with gout. Very uncommonly, rheumatoid nodules are present by themselves, without any other evidence for RA.

The exact cause of rheumatoid nodules is not known. There must be some factor beyond local pressure or injury, as nodules appear in less than 20 per cent of cases.

In some patients, treatment with methotrexate, even though it helps control joint inflammation, causes the nodule problem to get worse – and we have no idea why.

Nodules that are particularly irritating or unsightly may shrink following corticosteroid injection, and some can only be dealt with surgically. Unfortunately, they often promptly return.

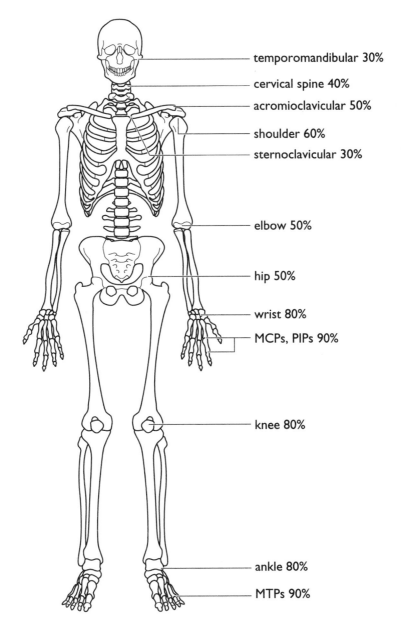

temporomandibular 30%

cervical spine 40%

acromioclavicular 50%

shoulder 60%

sternoclavicular 30%

elbow 50%

hip 50%

wrist 80%

MCPs, PIPs 90%

knee 80%

ankle 80%

MTPs 90%

Figure 2.1 Frequency of RA in the various joints

Because almost all patients with nodules have rheumatoid factor (RF) in their blood, RF may be involved in 'vasculitis' (inflammation of a small blood vessel) triggered by local injury from pressure. The body may react locally to the vasculitis inflammation, and the attempt at healing may result in a lump of scar tissue below the skin.

Nodules may eventually go away but they often persist after all other evidence of RA has been suppressed.

Rheumatoid factor

Rheumatoid factor (RF) is a protein that can be detected in the blood of most patients with RA. It's an antibody – a type of protein that is normally produced to fight off infection. In the case of RF, however, there is no obvious infecting agent, so we don't know what triggers the production of the antibody. Many different organisms, both bacterial and viral, have been suspected, but convincing evidence for any infectious cause has never been found.

RF is produced by lymphocytes, a type of white blood cell that collects in great numbers in the inflamed joints in people with rheumatoid arthritis. RF certainly plays a role in the inflammation and the damage in the joint, and elsewhere, that results. Its precise role is under study.

RF is found in the blood of about 60 per cent of new cases of rheumatoid arthritis, and these patients are called 'seropositives'. In general, people who are 'seropositive' right from the beginning are affected much more severely than 'seronegatives'. As the disease progresses, more and more patients change from 'seronegative' to 'seropositive'. Even then, though, up to 20 per cent remain RF-negative. It's quite possible that these patients have an entirely different, although very similar, disease. People who smoke cigarettes and have rheumatoid arthritis are more likely to have RF in their blood – and have more complicated RA than non-smokers.

RF is also found in other diseases, with and without arthritis, and in some 'normal' people. Clearly, rheumatoid factor has a lot to do with RA, but it is not the cause.

X-ray changes

The most typical change observed using X-rays is an erosion of bone at the margins of a joint. These changes can be seen in any joint that is inflamed long enough. Although a few patients are remarkably resistant to this development, 70 per cent of those who eventually develop erosions will show the first evidence of this within three years. In fact, one research study showed that this can happen by the end of the first year. This is the main reason why doctors tend to treat RA much more aggressively than they used to. We now realise that it's a lot easier to prevent damage than to reverse it.

How does RA first show up?

The sudden, explosive onset

Life for Mark, a 56-year-old security guard, was literally transformed over three days. This man who had never taken a sick day was suddenly unable to shampoo his hair, and could barely hold a knife and fork. Almost three dozen joints were swollen and painful – fingers and wrists, shoulders, ankles and toes. Even his left jaw (temporomandibular) joint was affected. He was stiff all day long, fatigued by four p.m., and only managed four hours' sleep at night because of shoulder and wrist pain. His weight had dropped 10–15 pounds.

By the time I saw him several months later, two additional pieces of information were available. Testing had revealed a positive rheumatoid factor (RF), and therapy with full doses of naproxen had done absolutely nothing.

Having discussed the issues with Mark, I initiated a programme to bring the condition under control as quickly as possible. I substituted prednisone for the naproxen and started him on weekly methotrexate. The prednisone, one of the most powerful anti-inflammatories we have, was for short-term control. The methotrexate would work more slowly but would eventually allow us to gradually taper off the prednisone entirely.

I saw Mark in follow-up two months later. He told me that after two days of prednisone he had been able to get his shoes on for the first time in two months. Except for slight swelling and tenderness in the right ankle, I found nothing on examination. He had no morning stiffness and had gained five pounds. He was back at work. His prednisone had already been lowered to twice daily. I gave him directions for further lowering of the prednisone, and an appointment in eight weeks' time.

About 15 per cent of cases 'explode' over a matter of a few days. Although not all the joints that will eventually cause trouble are

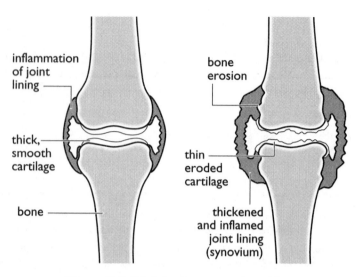

Figure 2.2 RA joint damage: early and late

involved in this first attack, there will be quite a number – two dozen is typical. They include both large and small joints, and especially the MCPs and MTPs. Similar joints on both right and left sides are involved. Morning stiffness and fatigue are prominent.

The gradual onset

About 75 per cent of the time – as with Sandra – the picture is less spectacular. A wrist becomes swollen and for some time it's the only problem. Or the person develops marked tenderness under the balls of both feet (the MTP joints), particularly when first getting up in the morning. Gradually, over several weeks to several months, more and more joints join the picture. Fatigue and morning stiffness make their appearance. It may take a year or so before the picture is clear enough for a definite diagnosis.

The gout-like onset

In 10 per cent of cases, RA starts off much like gout. A single joint, such as a knee, wrist or shoulder, suddenly becomes very painful, swollen and warm. Often the pain is so severe that the joint can't be used. Two or three days later, it's back to normal. After a month or so, another attack strikes, usually in another joint. As time goes by, the attacks become more frequent.

Gradually they are less and less severe but more and more frequent, and, instead of clearing up, the swelling and pain start to persist. One day, perhaps after a year or more, it becomes obvious that we are dealing with RA. This pattern is called 'palindromic rheumatism', and although it doesn't always turn out to be RA, it most often does.

Julie is a 36-year-old secretary. Nine months before I first saw her, she suddenly developed a very swollen, red and extremely painful left wrist. It felt, she said, as if someone had stuck a knife in it and was twisting the blade. She's right-handed and couldn't think what she had done to provoke this. For three days she had taken paracetamol with codeine 'by the handful' yet had very little sleep, and then, for no apparent reason, the pain and swelling had vanished. Two months later, the same wrist had the same pain and swelling, and the same outcome – gone in three days. One month later it was her right shoulder; for three days she had to use her left hand to brush her teeth. This was followed by three months free of any symptoms, and then her feet began to bother her. Walking, especially first thing in the morning, became very painful. The balls of her feet – the MTP joints – were the problem. Six weeks before I saw her she had developed swelling in several MCP and PIP joints. Pain and stiffness had settled into both hands and wrists. Pain in her shoulders awakened her at night, and her ankles became swollen. She was experiencing severe stiffness until noon, and was profoundly fatigued.

Julie's family doctor had already done blood tests. Rheumatoid factor was present, and there was no question that her palindromic rheumatism had evolved into RA.

I put her on diclofenac, an NSAID, but knew it wouldn't be enough. She was really hurting and I wanted to get control as soon as possible. I added methotrexate to the diclofenac, and saw her a month later. She was improved but still had a long way to go. I increased the dose of methotrexate. Today she phoned me. She was apologetic but firm. She had stopped the methotrexate; although I had given her an information sheet on the drug, and discussed it with her, she had read more about it and talked to some friends. She was afraid of what it might do to her in the long run. This fear of medication is common. Lists of side effects, however rare, are frightening. I tried to reassure her but I didn't push too hard. She has an appointment in two weeks. I expect she will be worse.

Palindromic rheumatism may clear up as mysteriously as it comes on, may continue indefinitely or, as in this instance, may evolve into very active rheumatoid arthritis, requiring aggressive action.

The non-joint onset

Very rarely, RA first appears in an 'extra-articular' (non-joint) site, with joint symptoms appearing months later. When it does, it usually takes the form of chest complications, and the patient is usually a man.

A friend and medical colleague asked me to see a patient of his. Oscar was a 45-year-old man who had been admitted to hospital two nights before. He had come in with what we call 'pleuritic pain' – a sharp, severe pain in the side of the chest that makes taking a deep breath very difficult. A chest X-ray showed an accumulation of fluid in the space around the lungs. The combination of pain and fluid accumulation is usually caused by an infection, but cancer or a blood clot in the lung can do the same thing. A good way of finding the cause is to do a 'pleural tap': a syringe is manoeuvred between the ribs and into the space around the lungs, and some of the fluid is collected and sent to the laboratory. In Oscar's case the fluid proved not to be infected but the sugar content was suspiciously low. This is rare, but my colleague is both well informed and bright. He ordered a rheumatoid factor test and it came out positive. That brought me on the scene.

Oscar by this time was quite comfortable and keen to get on his way. He had absolutely no symptoms of arthritis, so I didn't hold him up. I did, however, book a follow-up appointment. When I saw him two months later he had begun having joint pain, and within another month the diagnosis of RA was clear.

That was fifteen years ago. I treated Oscar with aspirin and started him on weekly gold shots, later spaced out to one each month. He's tried to drop the shots entirely on a couple of occasions, but each time his joints flare up. When that happens, I put him back on weekly shots until he settles down and is able to resume the monthly schedule.

I see Oscar about twice a year, to see how he's doing and renew his prescriptions. Visits are in the spring and autumn, which fits in with his work. He's a crop-duster, and his work takes him from coast to coast. As far as I know, he hasn't missed a day of work since his hospitalisation. If I didn't know he had RA, I certainly couldn't tell by looking at him.

How is RA treated?

Rheumatoid arthritis seldom goes away: 80 per cent or more of patients will continue to live with it. When its initial symptoms appear, it's impossible to tell who will do well and who will do badly. But we do know that joint damage occurs early on, and that we have only a very short period of time – a year or less – to prevent this damage with an effective treatment programme. In practice, this means that treatment is divided into two phases:

- an initial phase (preferably short) where RA is suppressed as completely as possible;

- a long-term surveillance phase where local complications of RA are spotted and dealt with before damage can be caused, and where major flare-ups are anticipated and prevented if possible.

A long-term contract

Treatment involves a long-term contract between physician and patient. Each must understand the other as fully as possible. Communications must be open. There will be times when contact is broken off because the disease is stable, but it must be re-established when necessary. And the patient must be able to judge when that time has come.

It's important for the patient to learn as much as possible about the disease, its complications and its treatment. Information can come from many sources – books, others with the disease and other health professionals including pharmacists. Arthritis Care is a valuable source of information (see the 'Useful organisations' section), and is the first port of call for anyone with arthritis. Its helpline can provide details of the many smaller organisations for particular types of arthritis.

It's also essential to be open and honest with the doctor. If you don't understand something, or you're worrying about something, ask. Doctors often assume that patients know more than they do, while patients are often afraid to appear 'stupid'. And if you are hesitant about taking a medication, or in fact are not taking it – for whatever reason – say so. Your right to refuse treatment is (or should be) recognised by the doctor. The fact that you are refusing shouldn't be taken as a challenge to the doctor's authority, and shouldn't cause him or her to refuse to treat you. There is almost always another way to approach a problem. If the treatment being recommended is truly necessary, more information or changing circumstances will probably enable you to accept it in time.

What tools are available to the physician?

Treatment can include any or all of the following:

- drugs – NSAIDs, 'second-line agents' (see later) and corticosteroids,
- physiotherapy,
- occupational therapy,
- social work,
- surgery,
- hospitalisation,
- monitoring the disease.

NSAIDs

Non-steroidal anti-inflammatory drugs are invariably the first 'class' of medication given, and one of the last stopped. They are described in more detail in the sections on drug therapy in Chapter 4, but a few generalisations are needed here.

There are a host of drugs in this category, including:

- salicylates (such as enteric-coated aspirin)
- ibuprofen
- naproxen
- ketoprofen
- diclofenac

- indometacin

- tolmetin

- the new COX-2 specific drugs (e.g. celecoxib, rofecoxib)

Whether it's an old-timer such as aspirin or a relative newcomer such as celecoxib, no single drug has ever been significantly better than another. But different people react differently, with regard to both good and bad effects. This means that a patient may have to try two or three different NSAIDs before deciding which one is best. 'Best' may mean 'most effective' or 'best tolerated'. If two drugs are equally good, the choice may boil down to 'most convenient' or 'cheapest'.

No NSAID can completely suppress rheumatoid inflammation. At best, perhaps 25 per cent of this problem will be dealt with – just enough to take the edge off. Because NSAIDs have both anti-inflammatory and analgesic (pain-killing) properties, it's sometimes hard to tell which of the two effects is helping the most.

NSAIDs are 'base-line' therapy – the first coat of paint. Once it's determined which one seems to be best, which usually takes a few weeks, it's time to add a 'second-line' agent, like a second coat of paint over the first. The second-line drug is taken in addition to the NSAID.

Five basic rules for treating RA

- Treat as soon as the diagnosis is made

- Treat to suppress all evidence of inflammation

- Fear the disease more than the treatment

- Treat the specific problem in the individual patient

- Use all available resources

Second-line drugs
As in psoriatic arthritis, second-line drugs are not as effective here as they are in RA. Methotrexate and sulfasalazine (and

corticosteroid injections) may help with inflamed peripheral joints such as knees and ankles but do nothing for the spine. The arrival of the 'biologicals' (such as etanercept and infliximab) has changed all that – they can make a huge difference in pain and, I hope, prevention of irreversible deformity.

Older, well-known drugs in this category include:

- hydroxychloroquine

- sulfasalazine

- gold compounds – both intramuscular (given by needle) and oral

- methotrexate (also known as amethopterin)

- azathioprine

In recent times, a number of others have been added:

- ciclosporin

- minocycline

- leflunomide

- etanercept

- infliximab

- adaluminab

All these drugs help suppress joint inflammation. As with NSAIDs, the discovery of the best one for the individual patient is a trial-and-error process. This doesn't rule out intelligent guesses, because the odds are better for some than for others. At best, a given drug will work well in about two-thirds of all patients, and have no major effect on the other third.

These agents are also called 'slow-acting drugs' because it may take up to six months for their full benefit to develop; even the fastest usually takes at least a month. Even if a drug works extremely well initially, as time goes by the benefit may be lost. This happens with all drugs in this class.

For many years, my usual practice was to try one second-line drug after another. If one drug didn't help after several months, or if it initially helped but later lost its effect, I would move on to the next on my list. This was acceptable for many patients, but for others valuable time was wasted; joints were being damaged right under my nose.

There is now proof that combining several second-line drugs (such as hydroxychloroquine, sulfasalazine and methotrexate) results in a better outcome, particularly in people with very aggressive RA.

Some of the newer agents – such as ciclosporin, leflunomide, etanercept and infliximab – also appear to work extremely well in combination with methotrexate.

In helping a patient choose a second-line drug or drugs, I attempt to calculate how aggressive that person's RA is likely to be, whether the 'window' until joint damage begins is fairly wide or just barely open. Relatively mild RA may allow for a leisurely trial of hydroxychloroquine; very painful and extensive RA, particularly in an older person with a positive test for rheumatoid factor (RF), calls for one of the stronger agents, alone or in combination.

Finally, for the very severely affected patient, one who has not responded to any of these conventional approaches, research is being done into the effectiveness of bone marrow transplantation. This treatment – which involves destroying the patient's own bone marrow blood cells with drugs, and replacing them with either donated or previously saved bone marrow cells – is essentially the same used in treating some forms of cancer. It is physically very difficult for the patient to undergo but the hope of a 'cure' may make the risk and discomfort worthwhile.

A number of people with severe autoimmune disease, including RA, have been treated successfully, but considerably more remains to be learned. Are there patient characteristics that can predict success or failure? What are the short-term risks of infection and death? What are the long-term risks of the arthritis coming back? Is it possible that the treatment itself may cause cancer?

Corticosteroids

Corticosteroids (also known as glucocorticosteroids or 'steroids') are synthetic versions of a hormone that is produced in the adrenal gland. This class of drug has incredibly powerful anti-inflammatory effects, but also has major side effects.

Corticosteroids come in tablets and in injectable forms, which may be given intramuscularly (into muscle), intravenously (into a vein), or intra-articularly (into a joint).

Because of the long-term risks of the oral form, it is wise to avoid it whenever possible. But low doses (5 milligrams or less of prednisone) carry very little risk, and in fact may help protect against joint damage. I use prednisone when the situation calls for it. This is usually when I'm starting a patient on a second-line agent. Steroids can be used as a 'bridge' until the second-line agent takes full effect or, later, as a supplement if the effect isn't quite good enough.

High-dose intravenous corticosteroids are sometimes used to provide short-term major suppression of RA until long-term treatment (that is, one of the second-line drugs) takes hold.

The risk with intra-articular steroids is very low and the possible benefit very high, particularly if a joint such as a knee is making it impossible for the patient to carry on. Benefits are felt almost overnight and tend to last for a long time.

Physiotherapy, occupational therapy and social services
A good example of what physiotherapists and occupational therapists have to offer can be found in Chapter 7. All are very helpful, particularly:

- to educate the patient about the disease;

- to teach the patient how to use joints without causing damage;

- to teach the proper role of exercise;

- to develop and teach programmes to get inflamed joints moving again;

- to provide splinting and cushioning to reduce pain and protect joints;

- to assess the home and the workplace and recommend changes or tools that will make functioning easier, less painful and safer;

- to provide an 'early warning' system, particularly if a problem arises that requires a doctor's attention.

The goal is to make the patient part of the treatment team. If the general principles of the treatment are incorporated into daily life, the course and the outcome will be much more favourable.

The help of social services can be crucial. Once RA develops, a number of issues can suddenly become major obstacles to recovery. Problems of short-term and long-term disability, income assistance and job retraining may seem too great to handle. Marriages can buckle under the stress of sudden changes in the patient's occupational, domestic and sexual roles.

Surgery

Surgery in RA has come a long way in the last 30 years. There is more extensive comment in Chapter 7 but here are some of the procedures used, with greater or lesser success:

- The most common type of surgery in RA is carpal tunnel release (discussed in Chapter 6). It is generally uncomplicated and very successful.

- Repair of ruptured tendons (almost always the ones that straighten out the fingers) is worthwhile and usually successful. It should be done as soon as possible after the rupture occurs.

- Finger-joint surgery can improve the look of the hand, but usually doesn't improve finger flexibility.

- Surgical replacement of knee and hip joints is usually extremely successful in restoring function and reducing pain.

- Shoulder surgery and foot surgery may help with pain, but are not as successful as knee or hip surgery in getting rid of pain or restoring function.

- Elbow surgery is in a transition phase. A new approach, using a three-part artificial joint instead of the older hinge prosthesis, is very promising for both pain relief and improved function. Whether the new elbow will hold up over time remains to be seen.

- In the past, surgical synovectomy (the cutting out of

inflamed joint lining) was often carried out in joints such as the knee. This isn't done much nowadays because

- the tissue often grows right back,

- rehabilitation is slow and difficult,

- infection is a real worry, and

- often the same result can be achieved with the injection of a radioactive form of yttrium, which burns and scars the inflamed lining.

Hospitalisation

Admission to hospital, particularly a hospital with a specialist rheumatic disease unit, provides the patient with a number of benefits under one roof at one time:

- respite from the physical demands of the household and workplace,

- the opportunity to rest painful inflamed joints,

- the skills of a physiotherapist and occupational therapist,

- the occasion to learn about the disease,

- the opinions of a variety of specialists,

- an environment where the effect of treatment can be observed, and treatment adjusted accordingly,

- access to a wide variety of diagnostic tests,

- assistance in addressing the many social, emotional and occupational challenges posed by RA.

Hospital admission is particularly helpful for the person who has only recently developed the symptoms of RA.

When hospitalisation is not a practical option, and often it isn't, therapy and other services may be available on an out-patient basis. Some professionals – in particular, physical and occupational therapists – assess and treat people in their homes. Indeed, this is often better than hospital assessment, as specific barriers to restoration of health and function can be identified in the home.

Monitoring the disease

One of the problems in treating RA is recognising when it's time to change the approach. It's too easy to check a patient briefly, mentally compare the status with what it was at the last visit, and continue the same treatment. Instead of words of encouragement and a prescription renewal, the patient often needs a major rethinking. Physicians' memories may be faulty, and patients who are used to feeling bad are often unaware of a slow change for the worse.

It's easy to monitor the progress of some conditions; with hypertension, for example, you simply put on the blood-pressure cuff and take a reading. There have been many attempts to develop a similar 'progress test' for RA but no easy answer has been found.

- X-rays are expensive, expose patients to radiation and record only major damage, after it has occurred.

- The duration of morning stiffness is a crude measurement of how well or poorly the patient is doing, as is the length of time it takes for fatigue to come on each day.

- Blood tests, and especially the sedimentation rate, are too inaccurate to be a basis for treatment decisions. It's true that rheumatoid factor (RF) often becomes negative in remission, but by the time that's detectable even the neighbours know things are better.

- A 'joint count' – an inventory of swollen and painful joints – is one way of keeping track over time.

- A number of questionnaires have been developed, and have been found to reflect very closely the activity of RA. The simplest of these, the HAQ, or Health Assessment Questionnaire, can be completed by the patient in minutes. It can help a great deal in determining whether a treatment is effective, or whether it's time to take a new approach.

What is the long-term outlook?

Ian became my patient 23 years ago. He was a policeman, 29 years old. For a year his sleep had been interrupted by shoulder pain, and he had been limping for the last nine months because of ankle and foot pain. Morning stiffness lasted four hours, but he continued to work. The rheumatoid factor test was strongly positive. I diagnosed RA, even though he hadn't yet had problems with his hands or wrists.

I started Ian on enteric-coated aspirin but he promptly developed a bleeding ulcer. (This can happen with any of the NSAIDs.) Like many people who develop this complication, Ian had no stomach pain to warn him. His stools turned black, standing up made him dizzy and his haemoglobin dropped. I stopped the aspirin.

Over the years, Ian has been on many NSAIDs and fortunately has never bled again. He has also been on low-dose prednisone for most of this time. Early on I started him on gold injections and for four years he did very well. Then gold lost its effect on him and I replaced it with penicillamine. Once more he did well, with an apparent remission for three years. Over the next seven years his treatment shifted back and forth between penicillamine and hydroxychloroquine, and his arthritis came and went. Control was erratic, however, so I switched him to methotrexate. These days I would start with methotrexate, which is much better than hydroxychloroquine and both better and safer than penicillamine. That was 15 years ago, and though he still has episodic flares – particularly in his knees, which settle down with cortisone injections – he considers that he is doing pretty well.

But years of rheumatoid inflammation have had an effect. He had to have two tendons in his left hand repaired because long-standing wrist inflammation had caused them to thin and rupture. Both shoulders have had surgery, and the joints have been replaced with metal and plastic. This relieved the severe shoulder pain that was the main reason for the surgery, but the range of movement in his shoulders is still very limited. This type of surgery has a long way to go before it will be as good as knee or hip replacement surgery. Finally, Ian has undergone fusion of two bones in his heel, in a mostly successful attempt to reduce the pain from a very badly damaged joint.

Fortunately, Ian has had a very supportive wife, and very understanding workmates. With modifications, he continued to work in the police department. In the past year, however, he did retire. He probably could have stayed on, but he was experiencing more and more pain in previously damaged joints. Now that he has stopped work, he has much less pain and fatigue. He has a bit of difficulty carrying out almost all activities of daily living – such as getting out of a bathtub and washing his hair – but there is really nothing he can't do.

The progress of RA is unpredictable but effective treatment does help slow the deterioration. In a minority of cases, there is total remission.

The outcome is likely to be poorer if rheumatoid factor is present from the beginning; if there are rheumatoid nodules; and/or if the patient is over age 60 when the disease first appears. However, the type of onset (sudden, gradual, gout-like or non-joint) is not an indicator of how the disease will progress.

The 'worst case' scenario is represented by a study in England: doctors looked back at 112 patients who had first been seen between 1964 and 1966. After 20 years:

- a third were dead,

- a fifth were severely disabled,

- a fifth were leading a normal life,

- almost a quarter had had major reconstructive orthopaedic surgery.

Disability risk has improved surprisingly little since then. A study in 2002 involving patients from nine NHS Hospital Trusts in England found that, of patients who had been working at the onset of RA, 29 per cent had quit their jobs five years later because of arthritis. This was particularly true for people involved in manual labour.

We have also known for some time that people with RA have a reduced life expectancy – up to six years in some studies. Deaths may be due to cancer (there is a very small increased risk of lymphoma), infection or, particularly, heart disease. A recent study based on the Norfolk Arthritis Register found that – in a group of patients whose RA had begun within the previous ten years – the death rate was roughly 50 per cent greater than expected, mostly from heart disease. This increase was primarily restricted to patients who were rheumatoid-factor-positive when the diagnosis was first made.

Most rheumatologists today feel very strongly that we can improve on the rather dismal results of the past. This is because:

- we realize that joint damage begins early (within months of the first symptoms),

- rheumatoid arthritis seems to respond to treatment better if caught in its early stages,

- we have a much wider, and more effective, range of drugs to draw on than ever before.

The challenge is to identify patients in the early stages of RA, and to ensure that they have ready access to specialist care – not just at the beginning but for as long as the disease is active.

Unfortunately, some patients are still more afraid of the treatment than the disease and shy away from second-line drugs. If the initial presentation of the disease suggests a milder course, this may not make much difference. But when the markers for more severe RA are present, patients need to understand the damage that may be done if second-line treatment is delayed.

Treatment may have other benefits. A recent study published in *The Lancet* and based on a 20-year follow-up of over 1,000 patients found that methotrexate – but none of the other second-line drugs used – seemed to eliminate the increased risk of heart disease death associated with RA.

Spondarthritis – inflammatory arthritis of the spine and extremities

This is a family of conditions that includes psoriatic arthritis, ankylosing spondylitis, the arthritis of inflammatory bowel disease and reactive arthritis (Reiter's syndrome).

Rheumatologists refer to this family as 'seronegative spondylarthritis'. 'Seronegative' simply means that the blood test for rheumatoid factor is negative, and 'spondylo' is a prefix that means 'spine'.

Members of this family of conditions share a variety of distinguishing characteristics:

- a unique pattern of arthritis in the spine and, often, extremities (hands and feet),

- inflammation of ligaments and tendons,

- occasional inflammation of the eye and heart,

- psoriasis in some,

- evidence of an inherited predisposition.

Compared with rheumatoid arthritis, this pattern of arthritis is likely to involve fewer joints, involve joints asymmetrically so that the 'twin' (such as the opposite knee) of an inflamed joint is not affected, and involve the lower spine, particularly the sacro-iliac joints.

Inflammation of ligaments and tendons, particularly where they attach to bone, is common and characteristic. The attachment points, in medical jargon, are 'entheses', and common sites of quite painful 'enthesitis' ('itis' meaning inflammation) include the back of the heel, where the Achilles tendon attaches, and the underside of the heel, where inflammation may produce a 'heel spur' (see Figure 2.3).

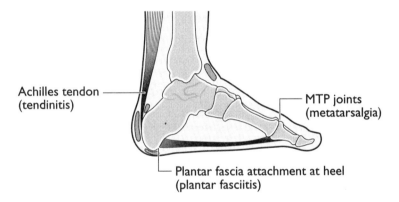

Achilles tendon (tendinitis)

MTP joints (metatarsalgia)

Plantar fascia attachment at heel (plantar fasciitis)

Figure 2.3 Common sites of foot pain

Inflammation of eye and heart tissues may also occur in these forms of arthritis, although this is fortunately infrequent. Eye inflammation is usually obvious, with redness and discomfort, and should be assessed by an eye specialist. Heart-tissue inflammation may result in a leaky aortic valve (so that blood leaks back from the aorta – the main blood vessel – into the heart) or in abnormal conduction of the body's electrical impulse that stimulates the contraction of the heart muscle.

Psoriasis, a chronic inflammatory disease of the skin, can accompany at least two kinds of spondarthritis – psoriatic arthritis and Reiter's syndrome.

Psoriatic arthritis (PsA)

Jim is a 31-year-old chiropractor with psoriatic arthritis. His hands are his livelihood. He has had psoriasis for 10 years. Because the rash is tucked away behind his ears and in the hair at the back of his scalp, not many people are aware of it. A close look at his fingernails, though, shows the telltale indicators. One is an accumulation of thick yellow debris lifting and irregularly separating several nails from their underlying beds. The other is the finely pitted appearance of many of his nails, as if a fine needle had pricked the surface, leaving dozens of tiny little pits in each nail.

Over the last four years the arthritis, which in his case involves mainly the end joints of his fingers (the DIP joints), has given him more and more concern. First one, then another, and now three of the end knuckles in each hand have become swollen and red. When the first one came on, it looked so inflamed that his family doctor put him on antibiotics, mistaking the arthritis for an infection. These knuckles are sore too, but not as painful as they look.

And it isn't just Jim's fingers. One by one, several of his toes swelled and became tight and shiny – what rheumatologists call 'sausage toes'. There were two toes affected on one foot, three on the other.

Generally, Jim gets by. He has some difficulty with fine finger movements such as buttoning and tying shoelaces and finds it difficult to open a milk carton. But before coming to see me, he hadn't bothered taking the NSAIDs his doctor had prescribed. He probably wouldn't have come except for two new developments – a tender right knee and a painful left thumb MCP joint. His arthritis had finally got his attention.

My examination confirmed the psoriatic changes in his scalp – fine silvery scales covered irregular reddish patches – and in the nails. The finger and toe redness and swelling were obvious. When I checked the knee, though, it was clear that the joint itself was not inflamed. The problem was with the tendon below the kneecap: it was very tender, particularly where it attached to the bone of his upper shin.

I prescribed an NSAID, in this case naproxen. My plan now is to see how Jim responds. I expect that he'll feel a significant lessening of his symptoms but that the inflammation will persist. If that is so, and if he agrees, I plan to add a second-line drug, in this case sulfasalazine.

What is psoriatic arthritis?

Psoriatic arthritis (PsA) is the arthritis linked to psoriasis. Although it has been around for years, it was only about 30 years ago that rheumatologists finally agreed that it wasn't just another type of rheumatoid arthritis (RA) but was unique.

One reason for the confusion is that PsA shows up in a number of different ways, one of which looks very much like rheumatoid arthritis. Another is that it wasn't really until 50 years ago that modern medicine began to look closely at arthritis in general. When that happened, people started to notice the differences in many kinds of arthritis, not just PsA. And this process of 'discovering' new kinds of arthritis isn't over yet.

Who gets it?

You have to have psoriasis to get PsA. Psoriasis is a very common chronic skin condition; it occurs in 1–2 per cent of white people. We don't know what causes it but inheritance plays a big role. Children of a parent with psoriasis are three times more likely to have psoriasis; if an identical twin has psoriasis, there is a 75 per cent chance the other twin will have it too. Its typical appearance is that of a reddish patch of skin covered with a silvery or yellowish scale. These patches (plaques) are of all sizes, and irregular in outline. They tend to occur over pressure points such as the knees and elbows. They are equally common in the scalp, behind the ears or in the navel. In fact, psoriatic plaques can be anywhere. They may be numerous, covering almost all skin surfaces, or found only after a careful search. They may come and go, and when they go the skin may regain its normal appearance.

As in Jim's case, psoriasis may affect the nails. This happens in just under half of all people with psoriasis (although the nails are involved in almost 90 per cent of PsA patients).

About 10 per cent of people with psoriasis develop PsA. If a careful X-ray search is made for evidence of arthritis (particularly if the sacroiliac joints at the base of the spine are X-rayed), this number can be pushed up to around 40 per cent, but most of the extra 30 per cent won't have symptoms.

Although psoriasis may start at any age, commonly in the late teens, the arthritis usually makes its appearance later – about equally in the 20s, 30s and 40s. I've said that you have to have psoriasis to get PsA. This isn't absolutely true, because in a small number of people (possibly as many as 15 per cent) the arthritis shows up first. The usual story, though, is that the skin rash has been present for a number of years, or (less often) that the rash and the arthritis develop together.

Finally, and this is very different from RA, the numbers of men and women with PsA are about equal.

Signs and symptoms that suggest psoriatic arthritis

- Psoriasis

- Redness and swelling at end knuckles

- Swollen, inflamed fingers and toes

- Tendinitis and enthesitis

- Back pain

What are its characteristics?

PsA has a number of distinct features. In some people one feature may dominate, in others, another. Features may be present in varying combinations, and the pattern may even change with time, so that the emphasis shifts. Characteristics that suggest PsA include the following.

Redness and swelling at the ends of the fingers
This is due to arthritis of the end knuckles (DIPs), and was the prominent feature of Jim's hand inflammation. Inflammation of the DIP joints is uncommon except in three instances – PsA, nodal osteoarthritis and (very rarely) gout. But in PsA the swelling and redness tend to involve the surrounding tissue as well as the joint. Not all DIP joints become inflamed, and those that do often develop the condition in sequence rather than all together.

Swollen, inflamed fingers and toes

This, too, happened to Jim. Here the inflammation is not confined to the joints – it spills over into the surrounding tissues. When I see fat, red 'sausage' toes, I start to look for evidence of psoriasis. Such inflammatory swelling of an entire finger or toe (called 'dactylitis') is almost always due to inflammation of the finger tendon, and in most cases that means psoriatic arthritis.

Tendinitis and enthesitis

'Entheses' are the points where ligaments and tendons attach to bone. Pain due to inflammation at an enthesis is very common in everyday life; 'tennis elbows' and 'heel spurs' are two examples. But in PsA, tendinitis and enthesitis are even more common. In Jim's case, the location was a bit unusual – where the tendon from the kneecap attached to the upper shin. Much more commonly, the inflammation involves either the Achilles tendon where it attaches at the back of the heel or the underside of the heel itself. This last location is where the tough tissue that protects the sole of the foot (the 'plantar fascia') attaches to the heel.

Back pain

Most people with psoriasis don't have back pain, but if they do it's identical to that of ankylosing spondylitis (AS). This type of back pain is characteristically worse at night, often awakening the person, and first thing in the morning. As the person becomes more active, the stiffness and soreness gradually lessen. There is another similarity to AS when PsA involves back pain – those affected are more than twice as likely to be male. This is quite unlike the equal sex distribution in other forms of PsA.

How is it diagnosed?

Diagnosis is easy if psoriasis co-exists with several red, swollen DIP joints, a swollen pink finger or toe, or a swollen knee, ankle or wrist.

In general, patients with PsA test negatively for rheumatoid factor (RF).

How is PsA treated?

Treatment of PsA and of RA tends to involve the same approach but with the major difference that PsA may not respond as easily to drugs that are usually helpful in RA.

- Oral anti-inflammatory drugs (NSAIDs) – rarely sufficient but modestly helpful.

- Traditional second-line agents (sulfasalazine, methotrexate, ciclosporin) may help with inflammation of the extremities (e.g. knuckles, knees) but seem to have no effect on inflammation in the spine.

- The newer 'biological' treatments (such as etanercept and infliximab) have been remarkably helpful – a real 'breakthrough'; they also seem to help control the psoriasis, too.

- Corticosteroids, by mouth or by injection, are useful, with the same qualifications we apply when we use them in RA.

- Occupational therapy and physiotherapy.

- Surgery if necessary, particularly when the hip or knee has been badly damaged.

What is the long-term outlook?

Two individuals I have come to know well over the years have had quite different experiences with psoriatic arthritis.

When I first saw Margaret a decade ago she was 46, the mother of two and a physician. She came to me with the following story. Psoriasis, mainly over the elbows and the back of the scalp, had developed when she was 21. At 34 she had a severe bout of neck pain for several months, and two years later an episode of severe right foot pain that also lasted several months. Its location, deep in the pad of tissue under the heel, as well as her recollection that it was very painful first thing in the morning and became bearable only after several hours of limping, convinced me that this was an enthesitis – in this case 'plantar fasciitis' (inflammation of the plantar fascia).

Six weeks before her first visit to me, the knuckle at the base of Margaret's right index finger (the second MCP) had swollen, turned red and become painful. Aside from scalp psoriasis and pitting of several nails, my examination turned up nothing of note. She had already started on naproxen and felt somewhat better, and I elected to keep her on it.

Over the next decade, she averaged three or four visits a year. Each visit would be provoked by something new happening – often the swelling up of one or two knuckles, with redness and pain.

In Margaret's case, the DIP joints have only rarely been inflamed – it is usually individual MCPs and PIPs. The swelling and pain tend to cool off gradually after two or three months. In only one case – the right ring finger PIP joint – has the inflammation caused any damage. In that case, the finger became 'stuck' in the slightly bent position. An X-ray showed no bone or joint damage; the problem is scarring of the ligaments and tendons around the joint. It is clear that, unlike RA, in PsA these structures are actively involved in the local inflammation. The spread of inflammation outside the joint itself is also probably why psoriatic joints so often look red, quite unlike those in RA.

On a half-dozen occasions, the visit was provoked by inflammation of individual finger tendons. This made bending the fingers to grasp an object, or make a fist, very painful and difficult. Sometimes, in fact, the swelling and pain would be so bad that the finger couldn't be bent at all. This problem usually melted away after I injected the swollen tendon sheath with a corticosteroid.

Once Margaret had a recurrence of her neck pain for several months, and another time she again experienced severe pain under her right heel. Twice her posterior tibial tendons (located on the inside of the ankle, just behind and below the bony 'bump') swelled. On several occasions she developed a fat pink toe, a different one each time. Walking was painful, so I had her shoes fitted with molded cushioning insoles until the inflammation went down.

And it did go down each time, usually within two or three months. She has been taking various NSAIDs – indometacin, piroxicam, naproxen – and they help with each flare-up. Unfortunately, she also gets severe 'gut-grief' with them, and has to take misoprostol (a stomach-protector). Eight years ago I started her on hydroxychloroquine and it seemed to reduce the frequency and intensity of her attacks. Three years ago I added yet another second-line drug, sulfasalazine, and I think she has done even better. I last saw her 18 months ago. She had just experienced a flare of inflammation of her right index finger DIP joint, her left index flexor tendon and her left *wrist. At my instruction she had taken a brief course of oral prednisone, and the flare had settled down nicely. There was little evidence of inflammation anywhere. I asked her to increase the sulfasalazine dose slightly. It must have worked, or her PsA is taking a holiday, because neither she nor her doctor has asked me to see her again.*

Margaret represents one end of the spectrum. Doug represents the other.

Doug was 47 when I first saw him eight years ago. Psoriasis had appeared when he was 37, and arthritis just three months before his visit. Within the span of these three months his right forefoot, at the base of the toes, had swelled and become red and painful. Three toes of his left foot had swelled, and his right knee was twice its normal size and painful. This was followed by pain under his heels that made it even more difficult to walk. He was forced to take sick leave from his foreman's job at an engineering company.

The intervening years have not been good. Doug hasn't returned to work. His feet have never resolved completely, and both hands, wrists, elbows and shoulders, as well as his right knee, have become inflamed, got better and worse, but never entirely cleared up. X-rays of his hands show erosions in several PIP and DIP joints, as well as the wrists. The toes show similar damage, and there are heel spurs. His grip strength, measured by squeezing a rolled blood-pressure cuff, is 110 with the right hand and 160 with the left (almost anyone without hand arthritis can achieve 300). He can do most things, but with a fair amount of difficulty.

Doug's gradual deterioration wasn't for lack of trying. He was faithful in taking whatever I prescribed, but most drugs upset him. Methotrexate and azathioprine caused quite severe nausea and vomiting. I tried intramuscular gold injections and they failed to improve him. At this point, it is difficult to know how much of his crippling — there is no other word for it — is due to the extensive damage that has been done and how much is due to ongoing inflammation. I am considering using one of the newer 'biologicals' — if I can persuade his insurance company to pay for it — and only wish it had been available years ago, before the damage had been done.

In general, although PsA causes long-term disability in some, this happens less frequently than in people with RA of similar duration. Nevertheless, after ten years of PsA at least 15 per cent of all patients are severely disabled. Probably an equal number, if not more, are in remission except for residual damage.

The same sort of treatment philosophy described for RA should hold equally for PsA. Because the outcome in any one individual can't be predicted, each person should be treated as aggressively as possible from the very beginning.

Distinguishing PsA from rheumatoid arthritis

Psoriatic arthritis may look very much like rheumatoid arthritis. For that matter, some people with psoriasis have RA – after all, both psoriasis and RA affect at least one per cent of the population, so it would be surprising if they didn't occur together. More often, though, one is confused with the other because both may involve the hands, and in particular the MCP and PIP joints. The diagnosis often rests on such features as the presence of rheumatoid factor and the changes seen in X-rays.

I was recently asked to see Anna because of this very problem. Five months earlier, she had experienced an explosive progression of pain, stiffness and (in the case of her arms and legs) swelling. The inflammation marched from her neck to her shoulders, and from there to her hands, wrists, elbows, knees, ankles and feet. Morning stiffness was prolonged and severe. Anna was 46 and was an executive assistant in a law firm, but had been unable to work since the episode had begun. Not only that, but she had real difficulty with such basic acts as attending to her personal hygiene.

Both wrists, as well as most of the MCP and PIP joints in both hands and both right and left MTP joints, were swollen and/or painful.

According to criteria set by the American College of Rheumatology (see the earlier section on rheumatoid arthritis), Anna had RA – a persisting, inflammatory, symmetrical arthritis involving hands and wrists as well as at least one other area, linked to morning stiffness.

But there were other features that indicated PsA. These included both right and left 'tennis elbows' as well as tenderness at the point on the right heel where the Achilles tendon attaches. In other words, Anna had enthesitis. She was also seronegative – her rheumatoid factor test had been consistently negative.

The most convincing evidence came from the past. She had been troubled with psoriasis as a teenager, although the only evidence for it currently was in her fingernails. In her early 20s, and continuing until the present flare-up, she had experienced periodic episodes of single joint inflammation that would persist for several months and then fade away. A number of DIPs and MCPs, as well as a wrist and a knee, had been the targets. This, then, was the background for her current flare-up – most unlike RA, but quite typical of PsA.

Rheumatoid arthritis versus psoriatic arthritis

	PsA	*RA*
Involvement of similar joints on opposite sides of the body	uncommon	usual
Involvement of DIPs	common	rare
Inflammation with joint redness	common	uncommon
Number of joints	fewer	more
Enthesitis	common	rare
Rheumatoid factor	in less than 5%	in about 80%
Rheumatoid nodules	absent	present in 20%
Sex ratio	equally affected	three times more common in females

---

Ankylosing spondylitis (AS)

Mike is 32 years old and works as a warehouse foreman for a department store. He was somewhat reluctant to come to see me. He had been living with his problem for so long that he felt there was probably little that could be done for it.

Mike was in his early 20s when his back pain started. He had twisted his back doing some heavy lifting and assumed this was the

---

The frequency of the various patterns of PsA

- 5–10 per cent look like Jim – primarily showing inflammation of the end knuckles of fingers and toes

- 5 per cent have low back pain dominating

- 20 per cent look like Margaret, with episodes of inflammation in relatively few joints in an asymmetrical pattern

- 70 per cent have persisting inflammatory polyarthritis, most like Doug, with characteristics of PsA, or, much less often, like Anna, whose arthritis is very similar to rheumatoid arthritis

---

cause. But when I heard his description of the pain, it was so typical that I felt it couldn't be anything but inflammatory. As he said, 'Nights are the pits.' He awakened regularly, around three a.m. each night, with a deep, aching pain that went from the small of his back down into his buttocks. Rolling over caused intense pain, and getting up out of bed each morning was an ordeal. He had to work himself into a sitting position, then slowly stand. The stiffness would gradually wear off by noon, and throughout the rest of the day, as long as he was active, he had no pain. It was only in the evening, getting up after watching television, that he was reminded of the misery of the night to come.

Over the years Mike's back pain had come and gone. There would be months when he wouldn't even think of it. But for the last two to three years it had been constant, and it was getting worse.

I asked the usual questions. Mike had never had psoriasis, or problems with diarrhoea or with a discharge from his penis. However, he did recall seeing an eye specialist five years ago, when one eye became red and painful. That got better with treatment and had never recurred. The other clue that I thought significant came up when I questioned him on other members of his family. It turned out that I had seen his mother, many years before, for a very swollen and painful ankle. When I later looked at my notes on her, I noticed that the ankle had settled down after several months, and that I hadn't been able to make a diagnosis. Maybe I could now.

When Mike stood, he had a slightly round-shouldered appearance, and the hollow in the small of his back was straight instead of curved. I measured his chest expansion with a tape measure. It was half of what one might expect. There was a similar shortfall when I measured the movement of his lower spine as he bent forward.

Mike's family doctor had made my job easy. He had ordered a sedimentation test, and the rate was markedly elevated at 55 milligrams per hour. X-rays had been taken of Mike's pelvis and lumbar spine; the lower two-thirds of the sacroiliac joints were partially fused, and several vertebrae showed bony spurs that looked as if they were trying to bridge the gap between them. Finally, although I certainly didn't need it to make the diagnosis, the family doctor had ordered a blood test for HLA (Human Leukocyte Antigen)-B27, and it was positive.

I spent quite a bit of time with Mike, explaining the nature of the problem and the role of treatment. I started him on indometacin, an NSAID, and arranged for a physiotherapist to show him a programme of flexibility exercises.

I've seen Mike once since. The indometacin hadn't given him heartburn, a possible side effect, and had given him a full night's sleep for the first time in years. He still had morning stiffness but it was much more tolerable. His main problem was fatigue. My measurements of his chest and back movements indicated an improvement of about 30 per cent. He was faithfully doing his exercises and had joined the Spondylitis Association. [In the UK there is the National Ankylosing Spondylitis Society.]

Ankylosing spondylitis (AS) is the most common type of inflammatory spinal arthritis ('spondylitis' means inflammation of the spine). In extreme cases AS goes on to become 'ankylosis' – that is, the normally flexible spine is transformed, because of persisting inflammation, into a rigid calcified column.

This member of the seronegative arthritis family is characterised mainly by inflammation of the spine, and only occasionally includes arthritis of the extremities. Psoriasis is absent, but some of the uncommon seronegative features – such as eye and heart inflammation – are occasionally seen.

Who gets AS?

Ankylosing spondylitis occurs in 0.1–0.2 per cent of white people (about one-tenth to one-fifth as often as rheumatoid arthritis). It's rare in black people, but much higher in some native North American groups. Men are three times as susceptible as women. It can occur at any age but the peak onset is in the late teens and twenties.

The 0.1–0.2 per cent figure is probably a minimum, because it's based on examination of people who were admitted to hospital. It is likely that there are many more cases, milder and undiagnosed, not in hospital. In fact, one Norwegian study turned up a frequency of just over 1 per cent, and only about one-fifth of these had ever been diagnosed! This could mean that AS is as common as RA.

What are the characteristics of AS?

Back pain with inflammatory features

This story is so typical that, assuming the doctor has time to listen to the patient, it should never be missed. Pain develops slowly, over months. The pain is so slow and insidious, in fact, that commonly several years go by before the diagnosis is even thought of.

The pain is 'rest pain' and comes on when the person is sleeping. It is at its worst when the person tries to move after being still for a while. It's made better by activity, often to the point where it's forgotten. It's often helped a great deal by NSAIDs.

All of this is in contrast to 'mechanical' back pain, which is what common-or-garden-variety low back pain (see Chapter 4) is called. The pain there comes on suddenly and is made much better by rest; NSAIDs do very little, and activity is associated with increased awareness of pain.

Inflammatory low back pain can be 'referred' to (i.e. felt to be in) the buttocks or even the upper backs of the thighs. Sometimes pain can be felt elsewhere in the spine – in the neck or between the shoulder blades. Chest pain, occasionally in the front in the area of the breastbone (the sternum), or coming around the sides of the chest from the back, is frequent, and can be quite severe. All these types of pain, like the low back pain, can be linked to enthesitis (inflammation at the site where ligaments and tendons attach to bone).

In AS, the inflammation is targeted on the spine and sacroiliac region of the pelvis, where the spinal ligaments and muscles are attached. This inflammation causes the pain, and also results in a very unusual form of reaction to inflammation. Unlike rheumatoid arthritis, where inflammation leads to erosion of bone, here new bone growth is stimulated by the inflammation.

Bony spurs grow out from the vertebrae of the spine at the sites of inflammation, tracing the course of the ligaments as they pass up and down to adjacent vertebrae. In extreme cases, these bony spurs completely bridge the gap between vertebrae, making movement impossible. If this happens throughout the spine, the individual stands and moves rigidly, unable to stand completely erect and unable to turn the head from side to side.

We rarely see people with AS ending up with 'poker spines' nowadays. Some experts believe that this is because NSAIDs help suppress the actual damage as well as 'cooling off' the inflammation. It's certainly true that before the 1950s – when phenylbutazone, the first truly effective drug for AS, became available – a bent, inflexible spine was accepted as an inescapable result of the disease.

Signs and symptoms that suggest ankylosing spondylitis

- Back pain with inflammatory features

- Occasional large-joint arthritis

- Occasional episodes of eye inflammation

- Rarely, heart inflammation

Occasional large-joint arthritis
This may happen in up to 20 per cent of people with AS. Hips and shoulders are the most common targets, usually in pairs (i.e. on both sides). Single-joint inflammation tends to be in a knee or

an ankle, and tends to be transient. Sometimes a jaw joint is affected but usually the joint is in the hip or leg. Interestingly, hip-joint inflammation seems to occur only in those who develop AS as teenagers, and then within the first ten years of the disease. It's very unusual for someone in his or her 30s or older get hip involvement.

Differences between men and women

In addition to the disease being less frequent in women (especially in the teen years), there are other differences. Women tend to have even more insidious back symptoms, and rest pain is less severe. On the other hand, it's much more common for women to develop arthritis in arm and leg joints, both at the beginning and later. Looking back, I think this was true in the case of Mike's mother. When I first saw her, ankylosing spondylitis was the furthest thing from my mind. In this I was undoubtedly blinded by the fact that she was a woman; at that time we thought AS was almost always a male disease. But it's also probable that her back symptoms were minimal and she didn't think twice about accepting them as 'normal'.

Eye inflammation

Attacks of iritis (inflammation of the iris) occur at some time in up to 25 per cent of people with AS. One eye becomes red and sore; vision is blurred and bright lights are painful. The attack subsides over weeks to months but, because the inflammation may leave scars in the area of the pupil, it's wise to see an eye specialist. Local treatment, and often long-term follow-up, may be important to prevent serious trouble later on.

Heart inflammation

Inflammation of the aortic ring – the tissue where the aortic valve attaches to the heart – may cause scarring and a consequent leaky valve. Because the electrical 'cable' that conducts the heartbeat is nearby, scarring can also cause a block in this impulse. It sounds terrible, and I spent a lot of time listening to hearts of people with AS before I realised that this is a very rare event; I've seen it perhaps twice in 30 years. The statistics say that it happens in about 5 per cent of people with AS.

How is AS diagnosed?

The most important clue to the diagnosis is the story of night pain and severe morning stiffness that improves significantly as the day goes on. Except in very early cases, physical examination may show that the spine and chest don't move normally, as in Mike's case. But this lack of movement doesn't necessarily mean that bony bridges have already formed; inflammation itself will interfere with movement. A good or excellent response to NSAIDs completes the picture.

The problem arises when the patient doesn't quite fit this pattern – usually because the response to treatment isn't as dramatic as expected.

Unfortunately, plain X-rays may not show any abnormality for up to ten years after the symptoms start, and nuclear isotope bone scans are often untrustworthy in AS. If a patient believed to have AS is not responding to the usual treatment, a CT scan is the best way of determining if there is sacroiliac damage. If this is positive, treatment should be pursued more aggressively; if negative, the patient's problem should be re-evaluated to see if there is another explanation for the symptoms.

Blood tests, and in particular the test for HLA-B27, are no help. A positive test for HLA-B27 is at least ten times more likely to be a false positive than a true positive.

Fortunately, most cases do fit the pattern, so there is usually no problem with diagnosis.

How is AS treated?

Non-steroidal anti-inflammatory drugs
NSAIDs usually make a big difference in ankylosing spondylitis. Unlike rheumatoid arthritis, where NSAIDs only 'take the edge off', in AS relief can be virtually total.

Phenylbutazone was the first of the NSAIDs available. It's still one of the most effective but, because it can cause aplastic anaemia (an often fatal condition where the body stops making blood cells), it is usually used only in those rare instances where all the other NSAIDs have failed.

Indometacin was the next NSAID available. It's quite effective but, because it can cause severe headaches when first taken, the

What is HLA-B27, and what does it tell us?

HLA stands for Human Leukocyte Antigen, meaning an antigen (protein) carried on the outside of white blood cells. The specific antigens we carry are inherited. These complex molecules are important in defending the body against infectious bacteria and viruses and other 'intruders'.

In the early 1970s it was found that, although one particular HLA, called B27, was found in only a small proportion of the population (about 10 per cent among Western white people), it was present in most people with ankylosing spondylitis (AS).

B27 isn't the only risk factor for AS, and most people with B27 don't develop the disease. But if one member of a family has AS, the risk for other family members who carry B27 increases to 20 per cent. And people who develop AS without carrying B27 usually have milder cases starting at an older age.

The importance of the discovery of the HLA-B27 link to ankylosing spondylitis lies in the questions it has raised about the ultimate causes of arthritis. Here is an inherited factor, a 'marker' for arthritis, that is intimately involved in the body's defence against infection. Armed with the knowledge that another B27-linked form of arthritis – reactive arthritis – can be triggered by a number of different infections, researchers are attempting to determine how this comes about. And because both systemic lupus erythematosus and rheumatoid arthritis also have inherited, and HLA, associations, the answer to that question may be the key to understanding many different kinds of arthritis.

individual is usually started on a fairly low dose and gradually worked up to a dose that controls AS symptoms. There is a slight risk of aplastic anaemia with indometacin, but it is rare.

Almost any of the NSAIDs on the market today is effective, but adequate doses must be used. The inflammation of AS tends to 'cycle'; that is, at times it will be relatively little and cause problems only at night and briefly in the morning. Patients should adjust the schedule of their pills to the disease: if symptoms are at a very low level, a single bedtime dose of

medication may do the trick. Indometacin is available in a
sustained-release form that gives 12-hour coverage, so it's
particularly useful in this situation. Sometimes symptoms
improve so much that regular NSAIDs are not needed.

After a period of time, many patients find that their NSAID
seems to lose its effectiveness. If they give that NSAID a rest and
switch to another for a month or two, they usually find that the
original medication, when begun again, is just as effective as it
was initially.

Second-line drugs
These have not proved as effective in the treatment of AS as in
the treatment of RA. Some – such as gold, penicillamine and
hydroxychloroquine – are useless. However, sulfasalazine and
methotrexate may be helpful in people with large-joint (non-
spinal) arthritis, and some of the newer agents, such as
etanercept, may turn out to be very useful.

Other drug approaches
Corticosteroid injections direct into the sacroiliac joints, under
X-ray guidance, may help relieve the pain of very active
sacroiliac inflammation. Some recent research suggests that
intravenous pamidronate (a drug used to treat osteoporosis) may
help where other drugs have failed.

Physiotherapy
This is (to coin a phrase) the backbone of treatment in
ankylosing spondylitis. In many forms of arthritis, physiotherapy
plays a supporting role; in AS its role is central. In the acute
phase of AS, physiotherapy can contribute a lot to pain relief and
to the restoration of normal spinal and chest movement.
Hydrotherapy in a swimming pool is one of the best ways to
achieve this. Once the acute phase is over, the hard part –
sticking to a regular exercise programme – begins. It's clear that
the eventual outcome of spinal movement depends on the
individual's commitment to a daily programme of exercise to
increase flexibility, strength and fitness. The most useful thing the
person can do is link up with a therapist who understands AS.
Once the exercise routine is learned, the person should get a
check-up at least once a year. Spine and chest movements can be

measured, and if there is deterioration the programme can be changed.

Occupational therapy (OT)
OT is not an issue early in the disease, except for advice on appropriate supportive furniture to ensure good sleeping and working posture. If ankylosis has occurred and the spine has become rigid, though, the advice of a therapist is more important.

Surgery
Surgery for AS is uncommon. When it is done, it's usually to replace damaged hips with artificial joints. The patient is invariably a young man, and the problem a combination of pain and severely limited hip movement. Short-term outcomes are excellent. Unfortunately, many patients will require further operations in the years to come, as the metal and plastic parts of the artificial hip wear down.

Education
In AS, as in other forms of arthritis, education is very important. Patients must know how to 'read' their bodies and must understand their disease. They have to be in charge of their medication schedule, and they have to understand the thinking behind all aspects of treatment, particularly the exercise programme. In many countries, particularly Britain and Canada, there are excellent national organisations for people with AS. They provide members with a variety of material (books, pamphlets, videotapes) as well as regular newsletters.

What is the long-term outlook?

For most patients, it's very good. Since 1947, researchers in Toronto have been following a large number of people with ankylosing spondylitis. At the 30-year mark they made the following observations:

- Disability developed primarily in the first 10 years, with little worsening in function after that time.

- Over 90 per cent of patients were coping with the demands of normal daily life very well.

- Pain continued to be a problem for many, but a third were pain-free.

Unlike with rheumatoid arthritis, there is no significant increase in overall death rates in AS. People should expect a normal life span.

Nowadays, with the benefits of NSAIDs and regular exercise known, there should be little disability from the arthritis unless there is hip-joint damage. Those who smoke should quit; the combination of smoking and a chest that doesn't allow full movement may lead to an increase in infections. If eye inflammation occurs and isn't treated, it may cause, over the years, problems with vision. Finally, those who have truly developed a 'poker spine' may be more vulnerable to spinal fractures, even with very minor accidents.

The arthritis of inflammatory bowel disease

When his doctor phoned me about Dennis, I knew I had to see him right away. Dennis was 28, and his problem was his right knee. Four days earlier it had become swollen and painful. I agreed to see him the next afternoon because the problem had many possible causes and the best way to get a handle on it as soon as possible was to get a needle into the knee.

As it turned out, I was none the wiser after the visit. Yes, after I had drawn off a sample of knee fluid and sent it to the lab I knew that the problem wasn't due to an infection, and that it wasn't a crystal arthritis like gout. But I drew a blank everywhere else. No other joints hurt, this had never happened before, he had no symptoms of any kind other than his knee pain and there was nothing in his family history that might suggest an inherited tendency. I put Dennis on an NSAID and arranged for him to come back in 10 days.

It wasn't a week later that I heard from his doctor again. Dennis had been admitted to hospital with severe abdominal pain. My first thought was that the NSAID had precipitated an ulcer, possibly even a perforation of the stomach. I was wrong. The admitting diagnosis was appendicitis, but once the surgeon opened the abdomen he found an inflamed segment of small bowel. Dennis had Crohn's disease. This was the clue I had needed to diagnose his problem: arthritis of inflammatory bowel disease. This is an arthritis that affects about 10 per cent of people with either ulcerative colitis or Crohn's disease, the two main types of inflammatory bowel disease.

Ulcerative colitis and Crohn's disease are conditions where the bowel wall becomes inflamed, ulcerated and/or scarred. These conditions tend to be chronic, waxing and waning over many years. The cause is unknown, but inheritance may be a factor.

Ulcerative colitis, which affects about 1 in 2,000, is a disease of the large bowel (the colon). It most commonly shows up as abdominal cramps with bloody diarrhoea. Crohn's disease affects slightly more people, possibly 1 in 1,500, and can affect both the small and large bowel. Its symptoms are similar to those of ulcerative colitis.

The arthritis of inflammatory bowel disease takes two distinct forms, one involving the arm and leg joints (peripheral arthritis), the other the spine (spinal arthritis). Either one may be associated with either of the two forms of bowel disease. It's possible for someone to have both forms of arthritis.

The peripheral arthritis tends to:

- be the more common of the two,

- involve large joints, especially a knee or an ankle.

- affect only a few joints (one to six) at a time.

- eventually settle down (half do so within six months),

- not cause joint damage.

Peripheral arthritis also tends to be an indicator of bowel inflammation, often showing up just before bowel symptoms appear or reappear (as was the case with Dennis), and improving when the bowel inflammation improves (either spontaneously or as a result of medical or surgical treatment).

Spinal arthritis tends to:

- be similar to AS in symptoms and X-ray changes,

- be present for some time (even years) before bowel symptoms appear,

- show up more as X-ray changes (15 per cent) than symptoms (5 per cent),

- be associated with HLA-B27 in about half the cases.

The spinal form does not usually improve with improvement of the bowel disease, unlike peripheral arthritis.

Both forms of arthritis may be associated with episodes of eye inflammation (iritis and conjunctivitis) and/or inflammation where ligaments and tendons attach to the bone (enthesitis).

How is it treated?

The peripheral arthritis is best treated by controlling, as completely as possible, the inflammatory bowel disease. This may not be easy. In difficult cases, local injections of corticosteroid can be very effective, particularly if the problem is only in a single joint, such as the knee. Sulfasalazine is a second-line drug that also has clear benefit, although it's no miracle cure. Methotrexate seems to help some patients. In a disease that has 'ups and downs', however, individual cases prove nothing. Proof requires a carefully constructed clinical trial and none has been done to date.

The spinal arthritis is more of a problem. NSAIDs such as naproxen or even indometacin can give good results, but may increase bowel irritation, and patients have to be monitored carefully for that complication. One of the new 'biologicals', infliximab, has been effective in helping to control the Crohn's bowel inflammation, and, although no study has yet been done, there is no reason to believe that it will not be equally effective in Crohn's arthritis.

What is the long-term outlook?

For the peripheral arthritis, the outcome is good. Disability and joint deformity are distinctly unusual.

The outcome in the spinal arthritis is similar to the outcome in ankylosing spondylitis.

Reactive arthritis (Reiter's syndrome)

I saw Don on the orthopaedic surgery ward. He was trussed up in a splint and bandages. He looked like hell. A 28-year-old farmer, he had been admitted the weekend before with the sudden onset of fever, chills and severe pain in the right groin. At that time, the pain was so bad that he couldn't bend his leg to slide his pants on. Putting weight on the leg was out of the question. An important piece of information came out at that time. Two weeks before, he had gone to his family doctor complaining of burning on urination and a yellowish discharge from his penis. He admitted to being what is euphemistically referred to as 'sexually active', and a tentative diagnosis of gonorrhoea was made. He was started on penicillin and, although the culture for gonorrhoea came back negative, the burning and discharge cleared up.

The orthopaedic surgeon, faced with severe pain in a single joint in a patient who had all the hallmarks of an infection, did the logical thing. He took Don to the operating room, opened up the hip joint and put in a drain. He started Don on intravenous antibiotics.

The reason Don looked like hell, and the reason I was asked to see him, was because he then went on to develop two fiery red eyes. 'Bloodshot' was an understatement, though Don did not complain of much pain. The big advantage in coming in late in a case like this is that it often makes more sense to a newcomer. Adding up the picture so far, we had evidence of arthritis, of urethritis (the discharge and burning) and of conjunctivitis (the fiery red eyes). I was pretty sure we had a diagnosis here – of reactive arthritis, or Reiter's syndrome – but I went for the icing on the cake, and found it. The roof of Don's mouth showed a large, reddened (and painless) area of ulceration, and the end of his penis, under the foreskin, was raw and inflamed. Finally, he had another feature that I've seen only a couple of times. The line of the hip incision was marked on either side by a weeping, crusting rash. It looked like psoriasis to me.

Hans Reiter, a German army doctor in World War I, put his name on this syndrome by describing an officer who developed infectious diarrhoea and promptly came down with arthritis, conjunctivitis (eye inflammation) and urethritis (inflammation of the urethra, the passage that empties the bladder).

Since then, a number of things have become clear: the condition is a systemic one, affecting more than joints; most, but not all, patients have the inherited factor HLA-B27; and the condition can be a reaction to any of a number of infections. Because of this, the term most commonly used today is 'reactive arthritis'.

Who gets reactive arthritis?

Reactive arthritis tends to strike young adults, most between the ages of 20 and 40; it's uncommon in the very young or the very old. This, and the fact that males are affected three times more often than females, has no ready explanation, because the factors that we know are involved don't discriminate by age or sex. The known specific infectious organisms that can trigger an attack of reactive arthritis can occur in anyone, as can the genetic inheritance of HLA-B27, which is present in 75 per cent of cases. The disease is fairly rare. Some 30 cases per 100,000 people are identified each year.

Only a handful of infections are considered to be triggers. These are, for the most part, organisms that attack the bowel and the genito-urinary tract. Some patients give a history of major symptoms of infection, some have had only mild symptoms and in some there is nothing to suggest an infection at all.

What are its characteristics?

Arthritis

Arthritis is usually what brings someone to the doctor. It is similar in its variety to all the other forms of spondylarthritis. In general, this means that it involves fewer rather than more joints, larger rather than smaller joints, and lower extremities (hips, knees, ankles) rather than upper extremities.

Swollen toes (dactylitis) and tendinitis or enthesitis are frequent. Back pain tends to come on if the arthritis becomes chronic. Joints are commonly very inflamed – red, hot, swollen and painful.

Symptoms of the 'triggering' illness

The patient may recall these symptoms preceding the arthritis by a week or two. They may include burning with urination, a discharge from the penis, cramps, diarrhoea and abdominal pain severe enough to raise concern about appendicitis. In many people such symptoms are so mild as to pass without complaint, and in about 10 per cent no symptoms can be recalled.

General symptoms
Feelings of severe illness are common: fever, sweats, loss of appetite, profound fatigue.

Psoriasis-like lesions
Eruptions of weeping and scaling skin may develop on the palms and on the soles, or the nails and skin may develop changes that look like typical psoriasis.

Mouth and genital ulceration and inflammation
Shallow, painless, inflamed ulcerations may be seen in the mouth and, in the male, under the foreskin.

Bowel and genital symptoms
Urinary burning and penile discharge may develop even when, as in the case of Hans Reiter's Prussian officer, the triggering event was an intestinal infection. The reverse is also true. A genital infection due to *Chlamydia* may provoke abdominal cramps and diarrhoea.

Signs and symptoms of reactive arthritis (Reiter's syndrome)

- Arthritis

- Symptoms of a triggering infection

- Symptoms of a generalised illness

- Psoriasis-like skin lesions

- Mouth and genital ulceration and inflammation

- Bowel and genital symptoms

- Eye inflammation

Not all of these occur together in the same person at the same time. Some patients (probably the majority) develop only one or two of the three characteristics that Hans Reiter described: arthritis, conjunctivitis and urethritis. These people are referred to as having 'incomplete Reiter's syndrome'.

In 1984 the Pope went to Canada, and celebrated a large open-air mass in Ontario. Many police officers from across the province were assigned to the event. Each was given a box lunch which contained, among other things, *Salmonella* bacteria. The food had been contaminated by a salmonella carrier. A total of 1,608 officers were exposed to this unexpected treat, and almost 30 per cent developed symptoms of infection.

Because this strain of *Salmonella* is a known cause of reactive arthritis, Dr Rob Inman and his colleagues in Toronto attempted to contact all who were infected. They sent out questionnaires and followed them up through the officers' family doctors. Of the slightly more than 400 who were infected, 27 (or 6.5 per cent) developed reactive arthritis: 9 cleared completely within four months, but at five years the other 18 were still having problems with arthritis.

Eye inflammation

Inflammation of one or both eyes is easily spotted and may be the first sign of the reactive arthritis. It has a tendency to recur, and because it can cause serious eye injury with the passage of time it's important that an eye specialist examine the patient. Long-term follow-up may be necessary.

How is reactive arthritis treated?

As with the other forms of seronegative spondylarthritis, it's the symptoms that are treated, initially with NSAIDs. Corticosteroids may be necessary, either by mouth or by injection into the joint. Second-line drugs are generally not used. However, if it looks as though the attack is going to be more drawn out, an agent such as sulfasalazine may be used.

Antibiotic treatment is still controversial. A recent research study suggested that antibiotics, given daily over a matter of months, may reduce symptom severity and shorten the period of illness.

The patient should be seen at least once by an eye specialist, because evidence of eye inflammation (though usually obvious) may be subtle and require a very careful examination.

What is the long-term outlook?

For most patients it is excellent. The acute inflammation in the joints usually settles down within weeks to months. But many people will experience some form of recurring symptoms over the years. These may simply be episodes of stiffness and soreness, particularly in the lower back. One patient in three will develop deterioration of the sacroiliac joints, visible on X-rays. Some will experience ongoing and quite disabling arthritis.

Eye and genital inflammation may have an even greater tendency to recur than the arthritis.

Systemic lupus erythematosus (SLE)

Laura is 23 years old and in her second year of medical school. I had met her briefly the previous year as a student in my clinical skills class. At that time I had been struck by the red, scaling rash on her face. It looked very familiar to me. So when she came to me just after Christmas and told me she had SLE I wasn't too surprised. What did surprise me was that she had made the diagnosis herself. So my job, after I had confirmed that she was right, was to determine how much she knew, what she feared and what she was prepared to accept.

The rash had begun a year before. It was red and splotchy, bumpy in some areas and flat in others, with a tendency to flake. It was on her forehead, her chin and the tip of her nose — but especially on the cheekbones just below her eyes. She had seen a skin specialist and had been given a cortisone cream. This had helped, but as the summer came on and she was outdoors more and more the rash worsened again.

A month before I saw Laura she developed arthritis. Her wrists and fingers were stiff and painful, and there was swelling of many knuckles. Her shoulders, knees and the balls of her feet were also stiff, particularly when she got up in the morning. It took her 45 minutes to loosen up. Her family doctor made an appointment for her to see me, and at her request ordered an ANA (antinuclear antibody) test. He also started her on an NSAID, ibuprofen, and this helped take the edge off the pain.

When I saw her, I learned a bit more. She had been experiencing mild hair loss all year. It wasn't enough to be noticeable to anyone else, but each morning she would notice a dozen strands of hair on her pillow. She had also been feeling very tired, her appetite was poor and over the year she had dropped about 2.3 kilos (5 pounds) below her usual 50 (110). She said she did not have Raynaud's phenomenon (see later), sores in her mouth, dry eyes, pleurisy or other chest pain. She was on no medication but the birth control pill.

Most significantly, her father had been diagnosed as having SLE some 20 years earlier. Knowing this, when arthritis developed, Laura went first to the medical sciences library and then to her family doctor. The requested ANA was positive.

I carried out a general physical examination. There were no surprises. Aside from some puffiness of her middle knuckles on all fingers of both hands, and traces of the rash on her cheeks, there wasn't much to find. This was one situation where laboratory testing would be important.

In SLE (also known simply as 'lupus') there is inflammation in many parts of the body. The joints are usually affected, which is why these patients come to me, but so are (or can be) many other areas – in particular, the skin, the blood, the kidneys, the nervous system and the tissues lining the heart and lungs.

SLE seems to be a disease of the immune system gone crazy. Antibodies (the proteins normally formed to protect the body against foreign invaders such as bacteria and viruses) appear to be formed against many of an individual's own tissues. These antibodies seem to trigger inflammatory reactions in skin, joints and all the other areas that are affected by the symptoms.

Who gets SLE?

A recent report based on an estimated 1.2 million people in the Birmingham area stated that:

- Roughly 1 in 3,500 people have SLE (1 in 2,000 adult women, 1 in 25,000 men).

- For every 25,000 adults, there will be 1 new case of SLE a year.

- The median age when people develop SLE (the age of onset) is 33 years in Caucasians and Asians, 26 years in Afro-Caribbeans.

- The frequency of 'new' SLE in Afro-Caribbean women is six times the rate in Caucasians.

- Afro-Caribbean women have more SLE complications.

Although sex and ethnic origin obviously play a role in SLE, occasionally it can occur as a complication of prescription drugs. Two well-known examples are procainamide, used for heart rhythm disturbances, and minocycline, commonly used to control teen-age acne.

What are the characteristics?

SLE has many faces. A rheumatologist usually sees a case that includes arthritis, a nephrologist sees one that includes kidney disease, a dermatologist sees one where skin rash is prominent,

Type of symptom	Present initially	Present eventually
General	75%	85%
Skin changes	50%	80%
Mouth sores	20%	30%
Arthritis	60%	90%
Pleurisy/pericarditis	20%	50%
Nervous system	25%	50%
Laboratory test abnormalities		
Kidney	45%	50%
Blood	15% or less	50%
Antibodies	95%+	95%+

and so on. As time goes by, a wider range of characteristics tends to develop. But in the individual patient, only one or two of these features may dominate and some patients never go further.

General symptoms

These aren't unique to SLE but are indicators that the person is 'all over sick', the state typical of, for instance, many severe infections. Fever is often part of this in SLE, as is a loss of both appetite and weight. But in SLE, possibly more so than in other types of arthritis, the symptom of overwhelming fatigue is striking.

> When I first heard about Roger from his family doctor, to say that I didn't accept his diagnosis of SLE would be an understatement. For one thing, Roger is male, and for another thing he is well and truly middle-aged at 49. He also lacks almost all of the general features of SLE. What he does have is:
>
> - Profound fatigue – this started a year ago. He loved to cycle and play tennis, and he suddenly discovered that he couldn't even climb stairs without stopping on the way up to rest. An effort like mowing the lawn would leave him exhausted for days. He had been forced to take sick leave from his job as a youth counsellor six months earlier, and he had come to believe that he would probably be unable to work again.
>
> - Profound depression, starting about the same time. It was so bad that he even considered suicide. Fortunately, he sought psychiatric help, and his depression, if not cured, was at least improved.
>
> - Stiffness and soreness, coming and going, in the knees, hips and buttocks. It occasionally wakened him at night when he turned over but for the most part it was tolerable.
>
> - Loss of appetite and a 10-pound (4.5 kg) weight loss.
>
> If I had seen Roger with only that information, I would not have put SLE anywhere near the top of my list. But, fortunately for Roger, he had a psychiatrist who was puzzled by the picture and followed up an astute hunch. He ordered a series of tests. One was the ANA test and the other was the anti-DNA test (see below), and both were positive. The ANA test told me that SLE was possible, and the anti-DNA test

indicated that a diagnosis of SLE was inescapable, even if he didn't have all the American College of Rheumatology criteria for SLE.

I put Roger on prednisone, 15 milligrams a day, and I saw him three weeks later. His life had been transformed. He felt wonderful. His energy had returned, he was back aj69

t work and he had resumed his tennis game. I outlined a schedule for reducing the prednisone, told him as much about SLE as I felt he could deal with in one sitting and made the first of a long string of follow-up appointments.

Skin changes

There are a number of ways that the skin reacts in SLE. One of the most common – seen in about a third of cases – is the *'butterfly' rash*. This is a reddish, slightly raised rash over the cheekbones (the 'wings' of the butterfly) and bridge of the nose. It may be itchy or slightly painful, and is often worsened (or first brought out) by exposure to sunlight.

The *discoid lupus rash* is less spectacular. It consists of bumps or small plaques with thickened scales covering them. These are chronic – that is, they persist for months or years. With time the central area of the plaques may become thin, flattened and white. This rash is common on the face, in the cheekbone area, but can also be found in the scalp or in other sun-exposed areas. Many people with discoid lupus don't have SLE, though some may, after many years of skin rash only, develop the systemic form.

The rash of *subacute cutaneous lupus* is halfway between the two already mentioned. Sunlight seems to affect it very much. This is the rash that Laura had. Some doctors feel that this kind of rash indicates a milder form of SLE but I don't think that's always the case.

Hair loss, or *alopecia*, is very common – it appears in about a third of cases – and seems to act as a marker of the level of activity. It improves as the patient improves and, as in Laura's case, seems to increase when the SLE flares. Hair loss is almost always diffuse, and not obvious unless carefully looked for. Bald spots are very uncommon.

Photosensitivity is a problem for about half of all patients. Exposure to sunlight causes a skin rash to develop or (as in Laura's case) get worse. In some cases photosensitivity extends beyond the skin, and can provoke a generalized flare-up of SLE. Because of this risk, I tell most of my patients to stay out of the sun. If this is unavoidable, I urge them to wear hats and long sleeves, and to use sunscreen.

Raynaud's phenomenon is a striking series of events that involve the fingers, and sometimes the toes, in up to half of SLE patients (as well as a large number of otherwise healthy people). With exposure to cold, a finger – one, several or all – goes white and loses all feeling. With rewarming the finger (or fingers) becomes bluish or fiery red (or both) and there is an intense burning sensation.

Mouth sores

Recurring painful ulcerations in the mouth or nose, and sometimes (in women) in the vaginal area, are fortunately not common. They tend to improve as the SLE improves.

Colleen and I have known each other for a little over 15 years. We first met in the hospital lab, where she works as a technologist. At that time she was 23. Almost immediately she became my patient. Her SLE came on quite suddenly. Initially it was a severe reaction to the sun – her face became beet-red and swollen, and stayed that way for three days. This was followed, over the next several months, by a series of symptoms that raised serious concern. She began to experience drenching night sweats, felt constantly feverish and was exhausted. Mononucleosis was the initial suspect, until her hands and feet became puffy and painful and she developed shallow ulcers on her tongue and the roof of her mouth. That, and the fact that she developed a typical 'butterfly' rash on her nose and cheeks, made the diagnosis obvious. The laboratory tests were, as expected, positive for SLE.

Colleen has been on prednisone almost all of the intervening years. For the first several years the daily dose ranged from 20 to 40 milligrams, with occasional bursts up to 60. Every time we attempted to lower the dose to a reasonable level, Colleen would develop more joint pain and new ulcers would appear in her mouth. Most uncomfortably, she also began having similar painful ulcerations in the vaginal area. Her rash and hair loss tended to have parallel flare-ups.

Ten years ago Colleen ruptured her left Achilles tendon. She had a few days' warning of pain at the back of her ankle, and then the tendon gave way. It was impossibly painful for her to stand on the toes of her left foot. With an ankle cast she healed, although she is still very weak on that side. The right ankle threatened to repeat the experience five years ago but it settled down before the tendon actually ruptured. This is a known but very uncommon complication of SLE. Prednisone is also suspected as contributing to the tendon weakness.

The only other area of difficulty has been periodic recurrences of painful bluish discolorations and occasional cracking of the skin at the tips of some of her fingers and toes. These, too – which I think are due to inflammation in very small blood vessels – seem to come and go with the other signs of her SLE.

What I haven't seen at any stage, despite careful searching, is any evidence of kidney involvement. Examinations of urine specimens, and blood checks for abnormal kidney functioning, remain consistently normal.

Colleen has done much better in the last few years – ever since I added methotrexate to the prednisone. Methotrexate, a drug that I use a great deal to suppress the inflammation in rheumatoid arthritis (RA), seems to have a similar effect in SLE. It has allowed us to lower Colleen's prednisone to a very low level – less than 5 milligrams a day – without any major return of her joint pains or mouth ulcerations.

Arthritis

This is one of the most common features in SLE. It occurs in the same pattern as RA – involving many joints, small and large, on both sides of the body, and in particular the knuckles of the fingers.

There are a couple of big differences from RA, however. The arthritis tends to be milder, responds to treatment more easily and does not result in cartilage and bone damage. Although the intense inflammation in the fingers may cause finger deformity, this is quite uncommon (less than 10 per cent). When it does happen, it's because of inflammatory weakening of the ligaments supporting the joints.

Joint pains (arthralgia) without obvious inflammation are as common as swollen joints. And, as Colleen demonstrated, tendons (particularly large ones such as the Achilles tendon or the tendon that anchors the kneecap to the upper shinbone) may become weakened and even rupture.

Pleurisy/pericarditis

Inflammation of the covering (the pleura) of the lungs is called pleurisy, and inflammation of the lining of the heart (the pericardium) is called pericarditis. Evidence of inflammation in these two locations is commonly found in people with SLE if it is looked for carefully, but the inflammation itself is usually without symptoms. When symptoms do occur, though, they can be very unpleasant.

The pain of pleurisy is sharp, 'like a knife in the side', on one side of the chest or the other, and is made much worse by deep breathing and coughing.

Pericardial pain can be very similar to the pain of a heart attack; it is usually described as 'heavy' or 'crushing', occurs in the centre of the chest and, like heart attack pain, may also spread into the neck or the arm.

Both types of pain generally respond quite quickly to treatment, which is usually prednisone. Sometimes inflammation in these locations is linked to small local collections of fluid in the spaces around the lung or heart, but it is extremely rare for these collections to cause trouble.

Inflammation can also happen within the heart and lung tissues, and in the heart such inflammation can damage the heart valves. When this happens, the damage may cause 'heart murmurs' (abnormal sounds detectable by stethoscope). Almost always, however, inflammation in these locations is silent, unsuspected and without serious consequences.

Nervous system

The nervous system includes the brain, the spinal cord and the network of nerves that travel throughout the body. Almost every part of the nervous system can be affected by SLE inflammation. The two most common problems, however, are headache, usually of the migraine type, and difficulties with concentration, memory and learning.

A number of other effects are not common but quite serious and are almost certainly caused by SLE. These include coma, seizures, stroke and nerve damage. Psychiatric symptoms, in particular severe depression, may dominate. In fact, depression seems to be the most common symptom of nervous system SLE.

Sorting out these problems, trying to determine if they are caused by SLE itself, by the treatment of SLE, or by some other factor, is very difficult. However, the more severe consequences often respond to intensive treatment of the SLE.

I was a bit surprised when, on New Year's Day, I was called by a colleague of mine about Mary Anne. I had seen her just three weeks before and she had been doing well. She wasn't now, and my friend had just admitted her to hospital.

Mary Anne was a 43-year-old mother of two and a part-time physiotherapist. I had seen her during her first hospital admission the previous October, when a diagnosis of SLE was made. At that time she had quite a few features of the disease, including joint pain and stiffness, Raynaud's phenomenon, a reddish rash on her face, fever and severe depression. She also had abnormal urine; testing showed both protein and red blood cells. Blood tests showed both a positive ANA and a positive anti-DNA, and a kidney biopsy showed 'diffuse proliferative glomerulonephritis' – one of the more severe forms of kidney inflammation. I gave her prednisone in a fairly high dose of 60 milligrams a day, and by the time she went home in mid-November she was considerably better. Just before Christmas I saw her again. She was still very tired, hadn't regained the 10 pounds (4.5 kg) she had lost, but the joint pains and rash had cleared. I added hydroxychloroquine and outlined a schedule for slowly reducing the prednisone over the next three weeks.

Now she was back, and the picture was quite different. Just about the time I was sitting down for Christmas dinner, Mary Anne developed a headache. It was dull and steady, across the forehead. She wasn't used to having a headache, and she certainly wasn't ready for this one. It kept getting worse and worse. Headache pills didn't help, and when her family doctor gave her a shot of pethidine (a very strong narcotic) it didn't work either. She began to vomit, and that's when she came to hospital and was admitted to the neurology ward. The next morning she developed double vision, and it was clear from examination that this was due to a problem with the muscular control of her right eye; the sixth cranial nerve wasn't working.

I filled her neurologist in on the background, and together we concluded that the most likely cause of both the headache and the nerve weakness was SLE. Mary Anne was given a series of 'pulses' of high-dose cortisone intravenously, and the effect was impressive. Within 24 hours the headache was gone, and by the end of the week her double vision had cleared.

That was ten years ago. Mary Anne stayed on hydroxychloroquine, and over the next few years she gradually discontinued prednisone entirely. There have been two occasions when I prescribed an NSAID for short periods because of a return of her joint stiffness and soreness. Depression has continued to be troubling, and she has been helped by counselling. But she has had no further evidence of involvement of the central nervous system, and her kidney function has returned to normal.

Kidney inflammation

Like just about every other part of the body, if the kidneys are carefully studied in people with SLE, some abnormality will usually be found. And, as with just about every part of the body, these abnormalities can be very serious but usually aren't.

Most commonly the abnormality shows up on urinalysis as microscopic traces of blood or high levels of protein. Blood can leak into the urine anywhere from the kidney to the bladder and the urethra (the passage from the bladder to the great outdoors). If the routine urine test turns up blood cells, I ask the lab to search the specimen again for 'red cell casts'. These are microscopic cylinders of red blood cells, and they indicate that the bleeding is coming from the filtering unit in the kidney called the 'glomerulus'. Inflammation in the glomerulus can also cause the filter to become extra 'leaky' – the 'holes in the sieve' become larger, and albumin in the blood, normally too large to pass through, gets into the urine. If too much albumin is lost in this way, it usually shows up as oedema (fluid retention), with puffiness and swelling – particularly of the ankles and feet.

Tests of kidney function (such as blood tests for creatinine and blood urea nitrogen) are usually normal. Both of these substances are filtered out of the blood by the kidney, and passed into the urine; if their level in the blood rises, it usually means that there has been a significant reduction in kidney function.

In the past, kidney failure was one of the major causes of death in SLE. It still is, but in the last 40 years treatment has made a real difference. Nevertheless, it's very important to be alert to the development of kidney inflammation, because there are no symptoms until the damage has been done. Testing of urine and blood at regular intervals is the best way to reassure everyone that no problems are developing.

There is still debate among doctors as to whether a kidney biopsy should be done in SLE patients who show urine abnormalities. The biopsy involves inserting a hollow needle through the skin of the back and into the kidney. A tiny core of tissue is extracted and studied under the microscope. The procedure is usually quite safe, but a very small number of patients require blood transfusions to correct bleeding after their biopsies.

When I was recently asked to see Marsha, it was to renew an acquaintance that goes back 26 years. She was 25 when we first met, and for most of the previous year, starting a month after the birth of her last child, she had been plagued by generalised inflammatory arthritis. She had none of the other features of SLE – no rash, no mouth or vaginal ulcerations, no anaemia and no kidney problems. But she told me about one episode that might have been pleurisy. To me her problem looked like RA, but testing showed the markers for SLE; there could be no mistake. For the next few years, arthritis was the main issue. I treated her with both prednisone and hydroxychloroquine, and she did extremely well. As usual, I adjusted the dose of prednisone to the minimum needed to suppress symptoms.

Then, after eight years, it became apparent that Marsha's problem truly was systemic. She developed more joint and muscle pain, and fever and night sweats. She developed an ulcer inside her nose that wouldn't heal. She became anaemic, and this was shown to be due to antibodies against her own red blood cells. Finally, after several months, her urine began to show red blood cells, red cell casts and protein. A kidney biopsy showed generalised inflammation of the kidney – the official report was 'diffuse proliferative glomerulonephritis', the same diagnosis given Mary Anne.

I increased the dose of prednisone and added azathioprine, a drug designed to suppress the immune reaction. Marsha responded. The joint and muscle pain vanished, as did her fever, and even the urine abnormalities improved.

I seldom saw Marsha over the next decade. She was followed up mostly by her family doctor, although she was also seen periodically by a kidney specialist, and I would get copies of his notes. From them I could see that she required very little in the way of prednisone to control her SLE symptoms. I could also follow, unfortunately, the gradual decline in her kidney function as reflected in her lab tests.

Earlier this year I was asked to see Marsha again. I learned that two years ago her kidney function had deteriorated to the point that she had to begin dialysis. Three times weekly she comes into the hospital for several hours to have a machine do what her kidneys can't. She is still working in the municipal planning office. She has no functional impairment (she needs no help either at home or in the office) and she has had no symptoms of active SLE for over ten years. This phenomenon is well known, as the symptoms of SLE often disappear when significant kidney failure develops. She remains on low-dose prednisone but we are going to try to slowly eliminate even this.

Looking back on the past 25 years, I often ask myself what I might have done differently. Even now our knowledge regarding preventive treatment of kidney damage is imperfect. I have always been concerned that an aggressive approach, using high-dose prednisone and immune-suppressing drugs, might cause far more harm than it remedied. Within the last ten years or so, some proof has emerged that cyclophosphamide modifies the downhill course. Had we known that at the time, we might have used it on Marsha, and risked some of the problems that drug can cause.

Blood changes

In the blood, there are three major types of cells:

- red blood cells, or erythrocytes ('erythro-' = red; '-cyte' = cell),

- white blood cells, or leukocytes ('leuko-' = white),

- platelets, or thrombocytes ('thrombo-' = clot).

In SLE, there may be reductions in the numbers of any or all of these.

Anaemia, or reduction in red blood cells, is usually not severe but can add to the general level of fatigue. Usually the anaemia is low-grade (mild) and develops in a manner similar to the anaemia in RA, as a result of inflammation slowing new blood formation in the bone marrow. Anaemia can also result from bleeding in the stomach or bowel because of NSAIDs.

Sometimes, though, the anaemia is quite severe and is caused by SLE antibodies directed against the blood cells, resulting in their premature destruction. This is called 'autoimmune haemolytic anaemia'. This process of antibodies attacking the person's own blood cells can also happen with white blood cells and platelets.

Leukopenia, or reduction in white blood cells, occurs commonly in SLE but is without symptoms. There are more than enough white blood cells to fight infection, though treatment with certain drugs may complicate matters and make infection a real concern.

Thrombocytopenia, or reduction in platelets, is much less common (possibly occurring in about 5 per cent of cases) and is usually without symptoms. Because platelets are important in blood clotting, if the reduction is bad enough it may cause easy bruising and even bleeding. This tendency to bruising is the first sign of SLE for some people. It usually responds quickly to treatment with prednisone.

Hélène has been my patient and friend for 30 years. A native of Paris who teaches French in the primary schools, she first came to me when she was 35. Even then, although it had not been diagnosed, she had had SLE for at least nine years. Her attacks of arthritis gradually became more and more frequent and widespread. Her fingers and wrists, knees, ankles and balls of her feet were variably swollen and tender. Fatigue had developed and, some two years before, Raynaud's phenomenon had appeared.

It was her family doctor who discovered that Hélène was anaemic. The condition was quite severe – her blood count was about half what it should have been. Investigations led to the discovery of antibodies directed against her red blood cells, and turned up a positive LE (lupus erythematosus) cell test which was at that time the best test we had for SLE.

I started Hélène on prednisone, and within a month her red cell count had doubled. She also regained 2.3 of the 4.6 kilos (5 of the 10 pounds) she had lost. I added chloroquine to her treatment.

Over the years I have continued to see Hélène, although not very often; the intervals are often as long as two years. These visits give me a chance to renew our acquaintance, practise my rusty French and keep an eye on her. We have both learned that the most common expression of her SLE is exhaustion. When it returns, and it does so at least once a year, prednisone is the only effective way to deal with it. She has also had recurring problems with a rash on her face, neck and arms. Now she uses a sunscreen whenever she goes outside in the summer. For a period ten years ago she awakened regularly with a severe cramp in the centre of her chest, a cramp that seemed to spread into her neck and left arm. An electrocardiogram and cardiac stress test were both normal, so I was pretty sure this was pericarditis and not coronary heart disease. The fact that her pain settled down with an increased dose of prednisone confirmed this.

Hélène remains on a low dose of prednisone most of the time. If it's stopped completely she invariably runs into difficulty – usually with fatigue. Her anaemia and her arthritis have never come back.

Antibodies

The main antibodies tested for in SLE (there are many, many more) are:

- antinuclear antibody (ANA),
- anti-DNA,
- anti-ENA,
- anticardiolipin (aCL).

These tests are used to help pin down a diagnosis of SLE. Whether they can also be used to look into the future of an individual patient is debatable.

The *antinuclear antibody (ANA) test* is very sensitive but not very specific. In other words, it will be positive in just about everyone with SLE – 95 per cent of all patients will be picked up. Unfortunately, so will a lot of other people, including those with other forms of arthritis, such as many that might superficially be confused with SLE, and many normal people. About a quarter of all 60-year-olds will have a positive test. So it is used as a 'screen': if it's negative and the patient doesn't have a rash that looks like subacute cutaneous lupus (see above), the doctor stops worrying about SLE. (People with subacute cutaneous lupus may be ANA-negative, but they are usually ENA-positive.)

The *anti-DNA test* is just the reverse. This test, which detects antibodies to the genetic material of the cell, is not very sensitive; many people with SLE will never develop a positive test. However, if the result is positive, the diagnosis is SLE; the test is extremely specific.

The *anti-ENA (extractable nuclear antigens) test* detects antibodies against a number of proteins in the cell nucleus. Some of these are very specific for SLE, whereas others can be detected in other conditions.

Anticardiolipin antibodies occur in some patients with SLE. Some (not all) people with anticardiolipin antibodies will develop the 'antiphospholipid antibody syndrome', which is marked by a tendency to form blood clots. These may show up in a wide variety of ways such as phlebitis (vein inflammation with blood clot development) and a tendency toward fetal death and miscarriage. A few SLE patients experience stroke and other neurological catastrophes, and anticardiolipin antibodies may be implicated in these.

It has been known for some time that one of the tests for syphilis (VDRL) was more likely to be positive because of SLE than because of syphilis. In fact, a false-positive VDRL became one of the diagnostic points in favour of SLE. We know now that the antibody responsible for this is an anticardiolipin antibody.

How is SLE diagnosed?

Diagnosis is easy if someone comes into my office with a number of SLE symptoms. Often, though, only one symptom is prominent at the beginning. Because I'm a rheumatologist, what I usually see is joint pain. If the story the patient tells suggests non-joint symptoms – a suspicious skin rash, sensitivity to the sun, severe chest pain, Raynaud's phenomenon – an ANA test is performed, which picks up at least 95 per cent of all people with SLE. An ANA test is done as well if the blood count or the urinalysis raises the suspicion of SLE, and on any young woman with joint pain. A negative result usually indicates that we're not dealing with SLE.

If the ANA test is negative but there are enough symptoms to raise suspicions, the ENA test should be ordered.

If the patient has only a few symptoms – such as joint pain – and the ANA test is positive, a diagnosis of SLE is hard to make.

Some patients need to be followed and tested for years before the picture becomes crystal-clear.

How is SLE treated?

SLE is a life-long disease. As in rheumatoid arthritis, the treatment of SLE involves a long-term partnership between the patient and the rheumatologist. Both need to learn how the individual's unique form of SLE affects that person, and how a variety of influences, including drugs, affect the disease.

Special attention needs to be paid to factors that might stir up problems – infections, reactions to drugs such as antibiotics, and exposure to the sun. A sunscreen with a protection factor of at least 30 is required if exposure to sunlight is unavoidable. Patients should get an annual flu shot, and those who have had their spleens surgically removed (one form of treatment for a low platelet count) should be vaccinated against pneumococcal infections.

In women, some drugs used in SLE may be harmful to a pregnancy, and birth control will be important if these are used. Birth control is also important during flare-ups, as pregnancy is best avoided until the disease settles down. But because oestrogens may play a role in SLE, low-oestrogen pills are recommended.

If the SLE is active, adequate rest is important – even to the point of taking time off from regular activities.

Regular check-ups, both physical and laboratory, are important to monitor SLE activity. This isn't always easy. It may be hard to tell old SLE injury from new injury, particularly in the case of the kidney, and drugs may cause side effects that confuse the issue. Blood tests may raise suspicions of an SLE flare, either current or incipient, but by themselves they are unreliable. There really is no substitute for an experienced doctor and a long-term relationship.

The drugs used for SLE are also used for other types of arthritis, and are discussed in greater detail in Chapter 7. Nevertheless, a few 'SLE-specific' points should be covered here.

NSAIDs

NSAIDs (non-steroidal anti-inflammatory drugs) are used in SLE much as they are in RA. They can be helpful in suppressing very mild joint symptoms but, as in RA, they often aren't sufficient on their own. However, they may help enough that only low doses of corticosteroids are needed to finish the job. Care must be taken not to combine them with more than 7.5 milligrams a day of prednisone, because the combination creates an increased risk of stomach bleeding.

There are two other concerns about NSAIDs. If there is a degree of kidney damage, NSAIDs may cause kidney function to deteriorate further. And sometimes NSAIDs cause symptoms that can be mistaken for SLE. Ibuprofen, in particular, will sometimes provoke fever, headache, neck stiffness and confusion. When the NSAID is stopped, these symptoms resolve.

Corticosteroids

Corticosteroids, like prednisone, were first used in the treatment of SLE in 1950, and the effect on survival was immediate and dramatic. It's not an overstatement to say that, in SLE, steroids are life-saving.

Fatigue, fever, arthritis and skin rash may respond to fairly low doses of 10 to 15 milligrams of prednisone a day. Nervous system involvement, severe blood abnormalities and active kidney disease may require much higher doses, although more than 60 milligrams a day is probably never indicated. It's a trial-and-error situation. Ideally, all of the drug is taken as a single morning dose, but if the flare-up is particularly severe the dose may have to be divided into two or three, and taken morning, noon and night. After the inflammatory flare-up is under control, the dose is maintained for a week or two and then slowly tapered down. As time goes on, most patients learn what a safe rate is, and how low they can go before a flare-up is inevitable.

For many patients, then, corticosteroids are an unavoidable part of SLE. The side effects and complications of these drugs have to be learned, and distinguished by both the patient and the doctor from the SLE itself. The section on these drugs should be reviewed carefully.

Antimalarials

These drugs, used to prevent and treat malaria, were accidentally found to be helpful in SLE of the skin. Since then, they have been used to treat other aspects of SLE, including joint pains, fever and fatigue, as well as the inflammation of rheumatoid and psoriatic arthritis.

Hydroxychloroquine is a particularly safe drug, but its maximum effect may not be felt for several months. It's not a 'first-string' agent; its use facilitates less use of other drugs, particularly corticosteroids. If hydroxychloroquine seems to help, it should be continued long-term, even if it seems that the SLE is in remission, or the SLE is likely to flare up again.

Investigational drugs

Drugs that have not been officially approved for use in SLE, despite years of experience, are called 'investigational'. Methotrexate, cyclophosphamide and azathioprine are some of the older drugs in this category – cyclophosphamide slows severe kidney inflammation and may help prevent the need for kidney dialysis. Leflunomide (a drug I use in RA) and mycophenolate mofetil (a drug used to prevent organ transplant rejection) may give me more choices if the optimistic early reports are borne out by further study.

What is the long-term outlook?

Systemic lupus erythematosus has changed from a disease that caused the death of half of its victims within five years of diagnosis to one where 90 per cent survive five years and almost the same number live ten years from diagnosis. Figure 2.4 shows American data but British results are similar: a group of SLE patients in Birmingham, followed up from 1991, had a 98.8 per cent one-year survival rate, 91.1 per cent five-year survival and 82 per cent ten-year survival.

There are many reasons for this change, but undoubtedly the discovery of corticosteroids, and their use in SLE, is the most important. It is likely that these drugs not only suppress symptomatic inflammation – arthritis, skin rash, pleurisy, mouth ulcers – but also reduce the number of people who develop important kidney complications.

The first five years are the most important. It's usually during this time that people find out what kind of SLE they have. Serious organ involvement, such as kidney inflammation, seldom develops after the first five years. Deaths that occur during that

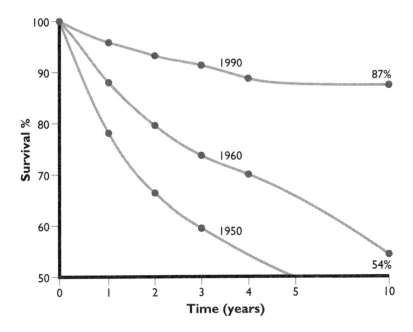

Figure 2.4 Survival rates in patients with SLE between 1950 and 1990

time tend to be caused by severe and uncontrolled SLE, particularly if the kidneys or brain are affected.

Predictors of a poor outcome

- Kidney involvement
- Nervous system involvement
- High blood cholesterol
- High blood pressure
- Need for long-term high-dose drug treatment
- African descent

SLE is a disease of relatively brief flare-ups separated by long periods of apparent inactivity. The only exception to 'what-you-see-is-what-you-get' is kidney involvement, where flare-ups can be quite silent. This underlines the importance of periodic blood and urine testing, over the long term. About 85 per cent of people whose kidneys are unaffected will survive 15 years, but this figure drops to 60 per cent if the kidneys are involved.

Severe involvement of the nervous system is also predictive of a poor outcome. Hypertension (high blood pressure) has been identified as a further factor and/or another reason for careful, long-term monitoring.

Treatment itself is not without risk. Long-term, high-dose prednisone or 'investigational drug' treatment may be complicated by a number of problems. Severe infection is one real worry. Similarly, treatment may lead to atherosclerosis ('hardening' of the arteries) by causing a long-term rise in cholesterol and other fats; there is some evidence that anti-malarials counteract this effect.

There may also be racial aspects to survival, even when the effects of socio-economic status are allowed for; in the West Midlands, as in the USA, non-white people have a poorer outcome than white people.

Polymyalgia rheumatica (PMR)

My father mentioned it in an offhand manner. 'I must be getting old', he said, 'I can barely make it down the stairs to breakfast.' The rheumatologist in me was suddenly awake. Even though I knew I was on thin ice (the jobs of being a doctor and of being a son should be kept separate) I asked Dad to tell me a bit more. Very severe stiffness had been waking him every morning for the past three weeks. He was stiff in the neck, the muscles over the shoulders and down into the upper arms, the buttocks and the thighs. He found it painful to sit up in bed and make his way into the bathroom. He had to inch his way downstairs, gripping the railing tightly for support.

By the time he finished preparing breakfast he could move much more freely and with less pain. What didn't make sense to him, however, was the fact that when he had finished breakfast and the morning paper he was stiff all over again. It took less time to get loosened up then, but the same pattern was repeated throughout the day; rest would bring on stiffness and activity would improve things.

These symptoms and the fact that Dad was 73 added up to a diagnosis of polymyalgia rheumatica (PMR). Reversing the usual order,

I referred Dad to his family doctor. He listened to the story, examined him, checked his sedimentation rate and reached the same conclusion. Then he started Dad on prednisone, and within days the pain was gone. 'I can't believe it! Prednisone is a miracle drug!' The testimonial was familiar, and added to my certainty that PMR was indeed the diagnosis.

That was over ten years ago. Dad is now off prednisone (he was on it for about five years, most of the time on very low doses) and his symptoms have cleared completely. I don't expect them to return.

Polymyalgia rheumatica, loosely translated, means 'many muscles hurt with rheumatism'.

We still don't know its cause, although heredity may play a role. Because it usually starts so suddenly, with flu-like symptoms, a viral cause has been sought, but none found.

Who gets PMR?

PMR is rare under the age of 50, but in the over-70s it's more common than RA, affecting about 3 in every 100 people. As is so often the case with arthritis, there is a sex difference – women are affected two to three times more often than men. It also seems to be primarily a disease of Caucasians living in the northern hemisphere.

What are the characteristics of PMR?

In most cases stiffness comes on suddenly and people can often recall the day and even the hour it started. Others experience a more gradual onset. Either way, the pattern is typical – symmetrical (involving both sides equally) muscle pain and stiffness in a shoulder and hip girdle ('shawl and shorts') distribution. Symptoms may spread up the back of the neck to the base of the skull, and tenderness of the buttocks after prolonged sitting is typical, but the muscles of the forearms and calves are spared. Sometimes stiffness is more localised, and when that occurs it's usually the shoulder region that hurts. The muscles may seem to be weak, but they aren't; it simply hurts too much to use them.

As in all forms of inflammatory pain, the symptoms grow worse with rest, and may even awaken the person at night. They are most pronounced first thing in the morning, and are made much better by movement.

There may be suggestions of a more general problem – fever and night sweats; loss of appetite, weight and energy.

A few people also have some joint swelling, at the knee or the wrist, most commonly, but it's usually mild and fleeting.

How is PMR diagnosed?

There is really very little else that looks like PMR. In the typical case, there isn't much question.

Sometimes, especially if the patient has joint swelling, the problem is confused with RA. Time and the response to prednisone help settle the issue.

Malignancy can look like PMR, particularly if the cancer involves the bone. A careful examination and a short trial of prednisone are helpful, as cancer pain doesn't vanish with prednisone. Low thyroid function and hidden infection are other things to be considered, as well as a bone condition – osteomalacia, due to vitamin D deficiency – which can be confused with PMR.

Signs and symptoms of polymyalgia rheumatica (PMR)

- Muscle stiffness in shoulder and hip girdle

- Usually abrupt onset

- Symmetrical pattern

- Pain with inflammatory characteristics

- Fever and fatigue

- Occasionally joint swelling and pain

- Spectacular response to prednisone

- Eventually, disappearance of symptoms

The most consistent laboratory abnormality is a high sedimentation rate, which generally reflects inflammation. In PMR it is usually higher than in other forms of arthritis. The saying in rheumatology circles is 'Both the patient and the sedimentation rate are over 50'.

But the most definitive feature of PMR is the effectiveness of prednisone. Symptoms literally vanish overnight with even relatively low doses, which would be most unusual for other forms of arthritis.

How is PMR treated?

Prednisone is not only diagnostic and therapeutic, it's also just about the only drug that really works. But in view of its possible side effects, it must be used with caution (see the section on corticosteroids, in Chapter 7).

The rule with prednisone in PMR is 'Go up suddenly, go down slowly' (see Figure 2.5).

What is the long-term outlook?

PMR does eventually go away. In some people this happens within the first six months, on average it takes about three years and, infrequently, it may take five years or more. Unfortunately, a few people still need to take 1 or 2 milligrams of prednisone each day to keep symptoms away, even after ten years, and I have had the occasional patient who, after a remission of a year or so, had a repeat attack of PMR.

The problem of giant-cell arteritis (GCA) and PMR

I had been following Sister Monica, a 76-year-old nun, for a little over a year. Her words, in a note she first brought with her, say it well. 'One day in March [two months earlier] I awoke aching from head to toe.... The nights were terrific. I was up six to eight times from the pain and got little or no sleep.... I'm a bit better now, but still excessively tired and I've gone from 124 to 106 pounds [56 to 48 kg]'. Her sedimentation rate was 95 (it's normally less than 20). She was anaemic, with a haemoglobin level of 94 (normal at least 125). She fit the profile of PMR perfectly. I started her on low-dose prednisone and she improved dramatically. By July a year later she was taking only 5 milligrams of prednisone and was symptom-free.

Two months later, things weren't going so well. Fatigue and muscle stiffness returned and two weeks before I saw her she developed a 'throbbing' tenderness over her temples. Four days later she noticed that her vision was blurred, and a week later she suddenly lost the vision in her left eye.

A biopsy of the left temporal artery (one of the areas that was so tender) showed the microscopic changes of inflammation that are typical of giant-cell arteritis (GCA). She was put back on a higher dose of prednisone. Her headache, stiffness and fatigue cleared promptly. Her left eye vision, unfortunately, did not return.

The case of Sister Monica is an example of something that happens occasionally – someone with PMR developing another, closely related, condition (in her case, GCA).

Most rheumatologists today consider that PMR and GCA are two ways that the same basic disease expresses itself. Both PMR and GCA occur in the same age group and both have high sedimentation rates and excellent responses to prednisone.

GCA (also known as temporal arteritis), though, is much less common than PMR. It's a condition in which inflammation of blood vessels of the scalp and head may cause:

- severe headache, usually in the temple region (this occurs in about 70 per cent with GCA);

- local tenderness, and sometimes redness and swelling, over the inflamed blood vessel;

- double vision, blurred vision or partial or total loss of sight (which is permanent).

Although less than 10 per cent of those with GCA will experience visual problems, this is the complication that is most feared.

In some patients, such as Sister Monica, the overlap between the two conditions is apparent. Indeed, about half of those with GCA also have the aches and pains of PMR. On the other side of the coin, if a biopsy of the temporal artery is done in a patient with PMR (even if there are no scalp symptoms) there is a 10–15 per cent chance that examination under the microscope will reveal evidence of GCA.

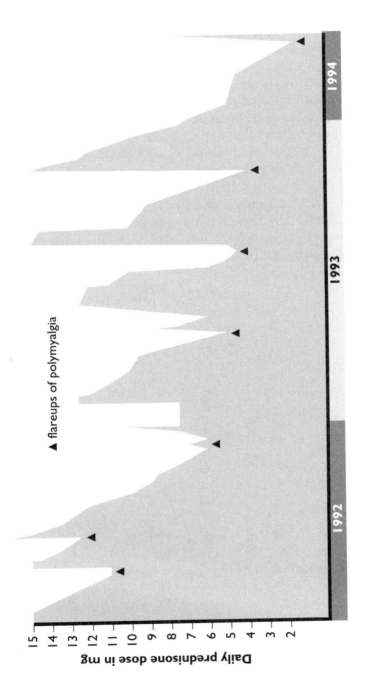

Figure 2.5 Controlling PMR with prednisone

What, then, is the risk of visual loss for someone who has only symptoms of PMR? There are no figures, but it's certain that the risk is very low indeed, far lower than the 10 per cent risk in GCA.

I've seen only two patients with PMR who suddenly lost vision in one eye. Both were on low doses of prednisone and had no symptoms of either PMR or GCA at the time.

My current practice is to tell my patients with PMR that there is a risk of GCA, that it is extremely small but it can't be eliminated. I tell them that if they ever develop sudden double vision, blurred vision or loss of vision they should take 'a handful of prednisone' (twelve 5-milligram tablets) and get to the hospital. Prompt attention may prevent permanent loss of sight in that eye and – even more to be feared – involvement of the other eye. If the second eye does become affected, it almost always occurs within a week of the first.

3
Arthritis Caused by Crystals

Gout

David, a 42-year-old accountant, spent the weekend in agony. From a vague ache at bedtime Friday night, the pain in his left foot had grown. When he awakened early on Saturday he couldn't bear to have the sheets touch his foot. To stand on it was out of the question, and putting on a shoe was impossible. By the time he hobbled into my office on Monday morning, leaning heavily on a borrowed cane, he hadn't slept for two nights, despite a dozen pain pills. He slipped off a heavy grey wool sock to show me his foot. It was puffy and pink from the instep to the toes. The area surrounding the base of the big toe was cherry-red, swollen, tense and shiny. When I held my hand a half-inch away (he winced in anticipated pain), I could feel the heat.

David had never experienced pain like this before. It was far worse than the fracture he'd had a month earlier, when his foot got in the way of a hockey puck.

David had no family history of arthritis and questions revealed no factors that might have provoked this attack of gout. But gout it certainly was. We proved it at his next visit by drawing from the toe joint, through a fine needle, a small drop of bloody fluid that revealed, under the microscope, the bright shiny crystals of the body chemical that causes gout. Before that, however, we had treated David with indometacin, an NSAID. It took several days before the foot was entirely normal, but by that next visit a week later the swelling, redness and pain had gone.

Gout is the arthritis caused by crystals of sodium urate deposited in the body as a result of long-standing abnormally high levels of uric acid in the blood. In David's case the crystals were in a joint.

Gout crystals also can be deposited in lumps under the skin (known as 'tophi') or in the kidney as kidney stones. It is important to keep in mind that gout is curable, and if treatment is started before joint damage occurs the long-term outlook is excellent.

Who gets gout?

Gout occurs in people with hyperuricaemia – elevated levels of uric acid in the blood. The likelihood of developing gout is directly related to both the degree of excess uric acid and the length of time that this abnormality has existed.

Gout is common – in Western societies it affects approximately 2 in every 1,000 people. It's usually a disease of adult men. In the age group from 35 to 45 years, 15 men out of 1,000 will be affected. The number rises with increasing age but the peak age for the first attack is 50.

Women do get gout but less frequently – one female for every seven males. The first attack is typically after the age of 60, and in women attacks may involve many joints at once from the beginning.

There is a family history of gout about 20 per cent of the time. Gout is also linked to a number of other medical conditions – obesity, hypertension, raised levels of cholesterol and triglyceride, hardening of the arteries and, possibly, diabetes.

What is gout like?

Acute attacks of gout are painful – more painful than almost any other form of arthritis. They come on suddenly, often without warning, sometimes after a few hours of vague discomfort. Single-joint attacks are the rule and any joint may be involved. However, the 'bunion' joint at the base of the big toe (the first MTP joint) is the most common. Doctors call this 'podagra' (literally, 'foot seizure'). After the big toe, the instep, the heel and the ankle are most common sites.

Untreated, attacks last from several days to several weeks. They may be infrequent – once a year or less – especially at the beginning. However, in the vast majority of cases, a second attack follows the first within six months to two years. As time goes by, attacks become more and more frequent – even monthly or weekly. Between attacks, at least in the early years, the affected joints look and feel perfectly normal.

Later on, if treatment of the high uric acid is not begun, about a third of attacks will be 'polyarticular' – involving a number of joints at the same time. The fever and chills that often accompany this kind of attack can make the doctor worry about the possibility of a blood-borne infection causing septic (infected) arthritis. This type of attack, though, responds just as well to treatment as the single-joint – 'monarticular' – attack.

Very occasionally, polyarticular gout may be less severe ('subacute'), and so persistent and involving so many joints, both large and small, that it's mistaken for rheumatoid arthritis.

Although not as spectacular, gradual joint deterioration resembling osteoarthritis may develop over time, even in a joint that hasn't been involved in previous acute attacks. It's particularly important for the doctor to be aware of this possibility, because it's entirely preventable with the appropriate use of allopurinol (see below).

How is gout diagnosed?

Other kinds of arthritis can be mistaken for gout. Other crystals can cause similar attacks, the most common being the calcium pyrophosphate dihydrate (CPPD) crystal of chondrocalcinosis (see 'Chondrocalcinosis', later in this chapter). Often, rheumatoid arthritis will begin with acute attacks of single-joint inflammation, but such attacks are usually less than 72 hours in duration, the big toe is rarely the target and in weeks or months the true problem is gradually revealed.

Finally, whenever any joint becomes suddenly inflamed, particularly if this is the first time, the possibility of a joint infection (septic arthritis) must be considered.

Gout can be diagnosed with absolute certainty only one way – by drawing fluid from a joint ('joint aspiration') and examining it ('synovianalysis') under a polarising microscope for the tiny crystals of sodium urate. Without such proof, the wrong diagnosis may be made and the wrong treatment started. If the attack is actually due to an infection, the wrong diagnosis may cost the patient the joint, if not his life.

Diagnosing gout from an abnormally high blood level of uric acid is a mistake. The level can be raised in normal people, especially those taking drugs such as diuretics and aspirin in low doses. And many people with acute gout will inexplicably have normal blood levels at that time.

If the patient is a middle-aged man with an acutely swollen big toe, an initial diagnosis of gout can certainly be made. But before a lifetime of treatment is prescribed, microscopic proof of the crystals' existence should be obtained.

Two other forms of proof, not as iron-clad as joint aspiration, are sometimes helpful. An X-ray of the foot may show evidence of bone erosion where uric acid deposits have worn away part of the surface of the bone. A 24-hour urine collection may show evidence of excessive uric acid production and excretion, and reveal the small number of people who are at risk of kidney-stone attacks.

What causes gout?

Uric acid is a normal body chemical, the product of a process known as 'purine metabolism'. It is derived both from the breakdown of protein in food and from the ongoing process of body tissue breakdown and repair. Some is reused by body tissues and some is excreted into the intestine, but most is disposed of by the kidneys.

In normal individuals, uric acid levels in the body remain constant because the rate of disposal by way of the kidneys matches the amount added each day through diet and tissue growth. But the process is out of balance in people who are either 'under-excretors' or 'over-producers'.

In under-excretors (most people who have gout) the kidneys filter almost all new uric acid, but a small amount is retained each day and over time more and more accumulates in the body. This has to go on for an average of 20 to 30 years before the first attack of gouty arthritis occurs. During this time, the excess uric acid is deposited in body tissues as crystals of sodium urate, because the blood simply can't carry that much uric acid in a dissolved state. An average person has about 1 gram of uric acid in the body. In gout the amount is two to four times higher, almost all in crystal form. In joints, crystals take the form of whitish deposits; under the skin, they form lumps or 'tophi'. Tophi are seldom detectable at the time of the first attack, but about half of all untreated patients will have them after ten years.

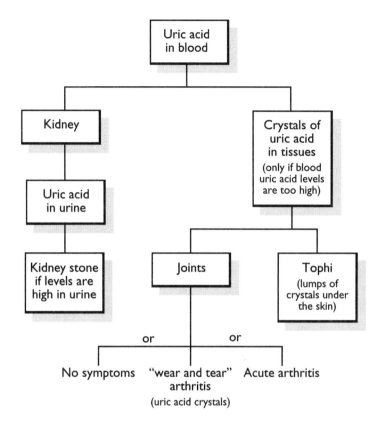

Figure 3.1 Uric acid: the cause of gout

This kidney defect is usually inherited, and the kidneys are otherwise normal. However, some drugs, particularly diuretics (drugs used to treat high blood pressure and fluid retention) can affect the kidneys the same way. If taken for years, they can cause sodium urate to accumulate, resulting in gout. Chronic obesity can have the same effect – not enough to cause gout but enough to aggravate the situation if gout already exists. Under-excretion can also be caused by long-standing kidney disease. For example, in the southern USA 'saturnine gout' is common. This kidney impairment is a result of chronic lead poisoning caused by drinking moonshine whisky.

Over-production of uric acid is a cause of gout in less than 10 per cent of cases. Research has shown that, in most of these, an inherited abnormality exists. The normally finely tuned process of uric acid production is out of control, and the rising level of blood uric acid no longer signals the body to stop making more. Most people in this category are otherwise normal, but sometimes excess production is due to abnormal cell growth, as in certain chronic blood disorders. Chronic alcohol overuse, particularly beer drinking, also seems to contribute to over-production, and may aggravate the situation in someone already predisposed to gout.

Because the amount of uric acid filtered by their kidneys is so large, over-producers are particularly at risk for uric acid kidney stones. An attack of 'kidney colic' due to such a stone may be the first sign of gout, occurring before the first attack of arthritis. And stones are not only painful; they can lead to kidney damage. It's important, therefore, to identify those who are at risk. This is done by determining the uric acid concentration in a urine specimen collected over 24 hours – the higher the result, the greater the risk and the more important early treatment is.

Why is gout so uncommon in women? It has to do with the blood's uric acid levels. In males, the level rises about 20 per cent at puberty. In women it doesn't; until the menopause, women's levels are consistently lower. Only if there is a major inherited abnormality, usually indicated by a very strong family history of gout, do high uric acid levels, and gouty attacks, occur in women during their child-bearing years.

What brings on a gout attack?

The sodium urate deposited in joints appears to be inert most of the time. However, for reasons not yet understood, newly formed crystals sometimes provoke a furious reaction within the joint. White blood cells, entering the joint from the bloodstream, attempt to engulf and digest these tiny crystals, much as they attack bacteria and other foreign materials. Urate crystals are, unfortunately, indigestible, and their chemical nature makes them toxic to the white blood cells. These cells literally explode, releasing their digestive enzymes and other chemicals into the joint and amplifying the inflammatory reaction. At its peak this response may involve hundreds of thousands of white blood cells. The result is a joint that shows all the classic signs of inflammation – swelling, heat, redness and pain.

Although we can describe the attack in cellular and biochemical terms, we still have little knowledge of the events that immediately precede it. Nor do we have a convincing explanation for the fact that, even without treatment, the attack eventually stops. We can, however, recognise some common situations in which acute gouty attacks occur. These include:

- Episodic excesses of alcohol and rich food

- Crash diets

- Local joint injury

- Hospitalisation, especially for surgery or heart attack

- The start of drug treatment to lower blood uric acid levels

Folklore links gout to high living, especially binges of alcohol and food. In this case, the story is true. The breakdown of large amounts of alcohol and protein in the body results in a brief but measurable rise in the normally constant level of blood uric acid. Alcohol in particular seems to be harmful – it not only blocks the kidneys' handling of uric acid, it also temporarily increases its production. (Alcohol does this to everyone, but only those who have accumulated sodium urate deposits will suffer attacks of gout.) It's thought that this 'blip' in blood level somehow affects the status quo in the joint, so that new crystals are formed, triggering the inflammatory response.

Crash diets, the metabolic changes associated with surgery and treatment with drugs that lower uric acid all cause similar 'blips', but in the majority of attacks we still have no idea as to the triggering events.

How is gout treated?

In theory we should be able to cure gout. We have extremely effective anti-inflammatory drugs; we also have drugs to lower the body stores of uric acid. In practice, however, the road to a cure can be long and difficult.

It is very important for the person with gout to know the purpose of each drug prescribed. They are not all the same. Some are to reduce the risk of an attack, some are to cut short attacks that do occur and some are to reduce the body load of uric acid. Until this high body load of uric acid is eliminated – and this may take several years – gout attacks can and do continue.

Treatment of acute attacks

Folklore (which in this case is true) recommends immersion of the painful part in ice-cold water. Fortunately, we also have a number of drugs that are very effective in treating gout. Most NSAIDs (except aspirin), when used in adequate dosages, work better and faster than older treatments such as colchicine, and without severe side effects. Treatment started at the first sign of an attack will end it in a matter of minutes to hours. If there is a delay of days, the attack will persist for days.

The 'gold standard' of treatment is indometacin, usually 50 milligrams every six hours at first, and then tapering off as the attack is controlled. Naproxen, piroxicam and other NSAIDs are alternatives. If taking medication by mouth is impossible, as when an attack occurs after surgery or in the presence of a bleeding ulcer, a corticosteroid ('cortisone') given intravenously, by intramuscular injection or even by direct injection into the joint, is the right choice.

For more on NSAIDs and corticosteroids, particularly regarding side effects and precautions, see Chapter 7.

Prevention of attacks

Colchicine can be used in low doses, daily, to prevent up to 75 per cent of recurring attacks. Aside from nausea, which may force a reduction from two tablets to one each day, there are remarkably few side effects. The only caution has to do with people with reduced kidney function, whose dose should be halved. Toxicity, which is rare, occurs when either too much is taken or a normal dose can't be eliminated from the body. The reaction takes the form of profound weakness, with nerve and muscle damage.

Regular doses of NSAIDs such as naproxen can also reduce the frequency of attacks. Unfortunately, neither colchicine nor an NSAID will do anything to reverse the continuing accumulation of sodium urate in body tissues or reduce the risk of insidious joint damage.

Prevention can also mean avoiding many of the things that provoke attacks, such as excesses of alcohol and (triggering) food at holidays, and crash diets afterwards.

Lowering of blood uric acid levels

Reducing the level of uric acid in the blood and gradually eliminating the body stores of sodium urate is the only way to 'cure' gout.

For many years, the only way to do this was with a diet low in protein. Unfortunately, such a diet was almost impossible to maintain and was only partially effective. Today such diets (termed 'low purine diets') are rarely used.

In the 1940s and 1950s, two drugs – probenecid and sulfinpyrazone – were found to promote excretion of uric acid by the kidney. They are still used today in some situations, such as the development of an allergic reaction to allopurinol. Unfortunately, for people at risk for urate kidney stones ('over-producers' and therefore 'over-excretors') these drugs increase the risk.

Today allopurinol is considered by most rheumatologists to be the best choice. The drug was developed in the mid-1970s as an agent to block the body enzyme that converts two other chemicals – xanthine and hypoxanthine – into uric acid. It does this very effectively, and with no new production of uric acid the old sodium urate crystal deposits gradually dissolve into uric acid, which is excreted. After several years the risk of further gout attacks diminishes, tophi disappear and the formation of kidney stones is stopped. Xanthine and hypoxanthine do not form crystals in the body and are easily excreted by the kidneys.

Allopurinol treatment should be started when:

- gout attacks are so frequent as to interfere with normal life;
- there is evidence that joints are being damaged by gout;
- tophi are present;
- urate kidney stones have been diagnosed;
- a 24-hour urine test has detected a significantly raised level of excreted uric acid.

Allopurinol may be used in situations where these criteria don't apply but the person simply wants freedom from future attacks. Some physicians begin the drug after a single attack, reasoning that an attack implies significant joint accumulation of crystals and inevitable joint damage. However, it is a lifetime treatment – if the allopurinol is stopped, the attacks will resume, often within the year.

In my experience, allopurinol is a very safe drug. There are a few things to know about it, however.

Rules for allopurinol

- Never start during an attack of gout

- Start slowly (I recommend 50 mg a day)

- Increase the dose slowly (50 mg every one to two weeks)

- Take enough to bring uric acid level below 350 micromoles/litre

- Combine with colchicine once or twice a day the first six months

- Once started, never stop

Indigestion is probably the most common side effect, and can be reduced by taking allopurinol with food. If ampicillin, a commonly used antibiotic, is taken at the same time as allopurinol, the risk of a skin rash is increased threefold.

Kidney insufficiency, common in older people, also increases the possibility of side effects on the usual dose of allopurinol. Some of these side effects (which can also happen to people with normal kidneys) can be quite serious, such as inflammation involving both the kidneys and the liver, as well as fever and skin rash. For this reason, allopurinol dosage must be reduced in the presence of kidney impairment.

There is another, more common, risk in starting allopurinol. We've seen that anything that causes a sudden rise or fall in blood uric acid levels (remember the effect of a rich meal and a few drinks?) can provoke an attack, and this includes allopurinol. Therefore, allopurinol is initiated with colchicine once or twice daily, with a supply of indometacin handy just in case. After the system has had a chance to adjust to the new routine (to be safe, many doctors wait up to a year) the colchicine is dropped.

If allopurinol is started while an attack is still going on, it prolongs the attack. The right way to introduce it is to control the attack completely with an NSAID such as indometacin, and start colchicine, to prevent a recurrence, once things have settled down. Only then should allopurinol be introduced.

Because obesity and chronic alcohol intake, particularly of beer, contribute significantly to the build-up of uric acid in the body, measures to correct both should be taken along with any drug therapy. It is very important to test for a high level of cholesterol (which is very common in gout) and to treat it if it is found.

Finally, drugs should not be used to lower a raised level of uric acid if there are no symptoms of gout. The person may never develop gout. Treatment may be not only unnecessary but also costly and perhaps harmful. It's better to see if there is a reason for the raised uric acid level and, if possible, deal with it.

Chondrocalcinosis (calcium crystal disease)

Donna is 65 and looking forward to spending the first years of her retirement pursuing her lifelong passion for bird-watching. I'm seeing her after an urgent phone call from the Emergency Room. She's been devastated by the onset, last night, of pain, swelling and warmth in her right knee. Although she was a bit more active than usual this past weekend, hiking the paths that border our local river, she's positive that the knee wasn't injured. This has never occurred before. Her health has always been excellent. Painkillers have only blunted her discomfort, but she is mainly concerned about the implications of the attack. Will this mean she has to change her lifestyle? Will she be crippled?

My initial assessment is acute monoarthritis. I run through the usual range of possibilities – infection, injury with bleeding into the joint, an unusual presentation of rheumatoid arthritis – but, based on probabilities and on the very sudden and intense nature of the attack, arthritis due to a crystal is high on the list. Gout is always a consideration, and Donna is sufficiently post-menopausal to be afflicted, but the syndrome of 'pseudo-gout' seems even more likely.

I aspirate the joint. A number 25 needle is thin enough that pain is minimal, and I take the synovial fluid to the lab myself. Under the microscope, the field is crowded with white blood cells – and many contain the telltale crystals of calcium pyrophosphate dihydrate. Back in the office, I review the X-rays taken earlier that day. A thin, milky line outlines the knee cartilages. I reach for my prescription pad.

Chondrocalcinosis (CC) refers to joint cartilage ('chondro-') becoming saturated with crystals of calcium ('-calcinosis'). The calcium crystal in this instance is calcium pyrophosphate dihydrate (CPPD). In most cases, there is no arthritis. But some people with this condition do experience episodes of acute arthritis that are indistinguishable from gout; others develop a picture indistinguishable from osteoarthritis.

Who gets calcium crystal disease?

The X-ray finding of cartilage calcification is common, but in most cases it means nothing. It's found with increasing frequency with advancing age; one study found it in a quarter of people over 85. It affects women twice as often as men.

On the rare occasion that it's found in someone under 50, it may be linked to an underlying disorder – most often hyperparathyroidism (abnormally high activity of the parathyroid gland) or haemachromatosis (a disease characterised by hugely abnormal stores of iron in the body). Chondrocalcinosis can also be inherited.

What are the characteristics?

I stopped Jim, a stocky 38-year-old laboratory technologist, in the hospital corridor. He was hopping along, one-legged, with the help of crutches. Ruefully he explained that he had come down hard in a weekend soccer match, twisting his right knee. I pushed the cuff of his trousers up and felt his knee. It was hot, swollen and very, very tender. Chondrocalcinosis was the furthest thing from my mind when, after some persuasion, he allowed me to aspirate the knee. But instead of being bloody, which I expected, the fluid was yellow and very cloudy. In short order we discovered CPPD crystals, found extensive chondrocalcinosis on X-rays of his knees and discovered that Jim's blood and liver iron levels were extremely high. Fortunately this condition, haemochromatosis, hadn't been present long enough to cause damage to the liver, pancreas or heart. Today Jim is a regular blood donor, which keeps his iron levels down, but his X-rays haven't improved. In fact, over the past 20 years a number of joints – his knees, elbow, ankle – have developed what I would call, if I didn't know the reason for the deterioration, osteoarthritis. Jim no longer plays soccer, but he is still a passionate hiker.

Chondrocalcinosis is without symptoms in most people with the X-ray abnormality. 'Symptomatic' chondrocalcinosis – the peak decade for symptoms is 65 to 75 years of age – can take two forms: acute and chronic.

Acute attacks

This 'pseudo-gout' may be indistinguishable from gout, except that the knee is the most common target; the wrist, elbow, shoulder and ankle follow. Attacks in the big toe are quite uncommon. The speed of onset is similar, as is the untreated duration: from one to three weeks. Most attacks occur without warning, but local injury or medical or surgical stress may precede them. Extremes of drinking and eating rich foods are not implicated. Involvement of more than one joint at a time is rare. Recurring attacks tend to come in clusters, but attacks themselves are far less frequent than gout attacks.

Chondrocalcinosis may be suspected as a cause of an acutely swollen joint in an older patient if an X-ray shows evidence of this. However, joint infection or even gout are equally valid possibilities. To be certain of the diagnosis the joint must be aspirated and the synovial fluid examined for crystals and bacteria. There are no blood tests to detect the condition.

Chronic arthritis

Chronic pain due to chondrocalcinosis may be mistakenly labelled 'osteoarthritis' (OA) because of many shared features – the pain and crepitus ('grinding' sensations or sounds) with use, a tendency to involve joints such as the knees and hips, and their appearance on later X-rays (which, because of advanced deterioration, may no longer show the telltale cartilage calcification). There are no figures on how often the mistake is made, but it is probably very common. Chondrocalcinosis may be one of the most important causes of OA. Its presence should be suspected when X-ray changes like those of OA are seen in joints that are rarely affected by OA – shoulders, elbows, wrists and the knuckles at the base of the index and long fingers – or when there is prolonged morning stiffness or too much joint warmth and swelling. Such evidence of inflammation can be so impressive that rheumatoid arthritis is diagnosed.

Chronic arthritis due to chondrocalcinosis is usually only slowly progressive, so most people cope with it well in the long run. Knees and hips, though, often eventually become so troublesome that surgery is necessary. Over all, however, when compared with people with OA, those with this form of chondrocalcinosis do much better indeed.

How does chondrocalcinosis come about?

A feature that distinguishes chondrocalcinosis from gout is that crystal formation occurs only in cartilage (see Figure 3.2). Calcium pyrophosphate, which is a common product of cell metabolism, seems to come mostly from cartilage cells. Why it combines with calcium to form CPPD is unknown, but there may be different reasons for different people. In most, the phenomenon is linked to ageing. In others, trauma is a factor. For example, chondrocalcinosis very often occurs in the remaining cartilage

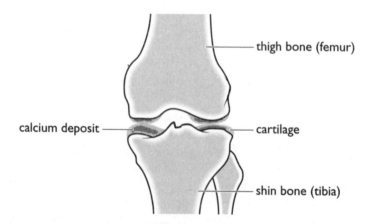

thigh bone (femur)

calcium deposit

cartilage

shin bone (tibia)

Figure 3.2 Chondrocalcinosis in the knee

The lost crystals

In 1679 van Leeuwenhoek, an early developer of the micro-scope, first identified crystals of sodium urate from a tophus (gout deposit), and in the 19th century Garrod found the same crystals clinging to a thread dipped in fluid from a gouty knee.

These lessons were forgotten, however. It wasn't until 1961 that Dan McCarty and Joe Hollander, using the polarising microscope in Philadelphia, rediscovered urate crystals in gouty joint fluid. They continued to look, and soon stumbled on the CPPD crystals in fluid from inflamed joints that were initially thought to be gouty. The chemical structure of this new crystal was worked out. Finally, the link was made between these crystals and the X-ray diagnosis of chondrocalcinosis.

---

after surgical removal of a torn knee cartilage. The excessive weight load borne by the cartilage that remains seems to be the culprit. In some cases, the chemical environment of the cartilage – high levels of calcium (in hyperparathyroidism) or iron (in haemachromatosis) – somehow favours the formation of CPPD crystals.

As with gout, we don't clearly understand what provokes attacks of pseudo-gout. Shedding of crystals into the joint space from their normally safe location deep in cartilage may be caused by local injury when the attack is linked to definite joint trauma, or to infection inside the joint, but doesn't explain attacks that come on with hospitalisation for surgery or heart attack. Once crystals appear in the joint, however, the same sort of reaction found in gout develops in a pseudo-gout attack.

How is it treated?

Acute attacks are dealt with much as attacks of true gout are – with NSAIDs such as indometacin or naproxen, or with cortico-steroid injection. The latter is often preferable, especially if an easy-to-inject joint, such as a knee, is the target. Not only does this ensure that a very potent drug is placed in precisely the right place, it also avoids the risk of NSAID side effects. NSAID complications, such as fluid retention, worsening of chronic kidney insufficiency, or bleeding of a stomach or duodenal ulcer, are much more frequent in older patients, the same people who develop chondrocalcinosis.

People with chronic chondrocalcinosis arthritis, particularly if there is a major inflammatory component or a tendency to acute attacks, are frequently placed on regular daily doses of an NSAID. In those over 65, drugs that protect against stomach bleeding may be prescribed as well, and side effects should be monitored even more carefully. Simple painkillers such as paracetamol are often adequate, and consultation with a physiotherapist is worthwhile.

Asymptomatic patients (those who show X-ray evidence of calcification but don't have pain) do not benefit from treatment. No way has yet been devised to reduce the burden of calcium crystallisation. Even where an underlying disorder has been discovered and treated effectively, chondrocalcinosis will persist.

4
Non-inflammatory Arthritis

Osteoarthritis

Osteoarthritis (OA) is sometimes called 'degenerative joint disease' or 'osteoarthrosis'. It's the most common type of arthritis, yet technically speaking it isn't 'arthritis' at all, because '-itis' means inflammation and OA usually has very little to do with inflammation. It isn't even a single disease. The best definition is that osteoarthritis is what happens when joint cartilage fails.

Here are four examples of what we call osteoarthritis, each quite different from the others. The four are chosen because they cover the most common and important varieties. Although OA can be found in any joint, it seems to affect primarily four regions – the knees, hips, hands and spine.

Example 1 – Osteoarthritis of the knee

Catherine is now 69 years old. She and her husband have run a gift shop in a small summer resort town for the past 30 years. I saw her last nine years ago. The problem was the same then as now – her knees. She really doesn't remember when they first began to bother her but it was at least 15 years ago. She has never had a severe flare-up of pain or swelling. She doesn't recall any injury to her knees, and she has never had arthritis anywhere else. She has always been somewhat overweight but is not obese.

'My knees still aren't much trouble. I really don't have any pain unless I stand or walk a lot. They don't hurt at night. When I first get up in the morning they're a bit stiff, but they're OK after a few minutes. I do have to be careful going down stairs. They don't feel very steady and I worry that they're going to give way on me. When I go out, I use my cane all the time. I know you told me to start using one after my last visit, but I was too proud for a long time. Canes are for old people. But I started to worry about falling and now I always use

it. I wish I'd done it before. The cane does help with the pain, and I can get about much better.

'I tried taking ibuprofen [an NSAID] but I didn't notice that it made much difference. Now, if my knees ache, I just take a couple of paracetamol. They do swell some, especially if I do a lot of walking, but I haven't noticed that they're very warm. I guess the reason I wanted to see you again is to find out if there's something else I should be doing.'

Catherine is dramatically 'knock-kneed'; when she stands, her knees touch and her feet are at least 30cm (12 inches) apart. Her knees aren't fully straightened out, either, which means she has to keep her hips slightly bent to stand straight. I go over her knees as she lies on the examining table. They are slightly swollen but cool to the touch. The swelling is partly due to an accumulation of fluid inside the knee joint, but some is a result of new bone that has grown up along the outside of the joint as part of the healing process. I bend her knees, each in turn. My left hand, cupping the kneecap, can feel a rough grinding sensation. I can almost see the roughened, deeply pitted surfaces of the cartilage. The knees are about 15 degrees from lying flat on the table, and I can only bend them to just past 90 degrees. I'm pretty sure the X-rays will show that new bone growth is interfering with full movement. With the legs resting as flat as possible on the table, I push on the inside of each knee. I can almost straighten out the 'knock-knee' deformity. This means that there has been a collapse of the outer half of the knee joint – the 'lateral joint compartment' – probably because the cartilage there has disappeared.

Another thing I notice is that her quadriceps muscles (the muscles on the front of the thigh) are much smaller and weaker than they should be. I'm pretty sure they can be strengthened by exercise. That will do a lot to help support and protect the knees, and even slow the wearing-out process. This type of exercise is the single most important thing that Catherine can do to reduce the pain.

We spend the rest of the time talking about whether she should be seeing an orthopaedic surgeon. Total knee replacement surgery, with metal-and-plastic artificial knees, has come a long way, and is now an extremely good choice for many people. But here there isn't a strong argument for surgery; pain isn't a big problem and her lifestyle is not significantly curtailed. She would do far better with a referral to a good physiotherapist, who could provide:

- a regular quadriceps-strengthening programme,

- *a programme of leg stretching,*

- *instruction in protection of the joint,*

- *assessment and advice regarding footwear,*

- *advice on a fitness programme that avoids abusing the knees.*

Then, if and when pain or disability reaches the point where surgery is appropriate, she'll get a better result.

Osteoarthritis of the knee is one of the most common forms of OA. It occurs in about 10 per cent of all people over 65, and in about 2 per cent of all adults.

Catherine is typical in many respects. She is a woman and she is in the older age group. Aside from her being somewhat over-weight (a risk factor for knee OA), there are no obvious reasons why her knees should be affected. She has surprisingly little pain despite the appearance of her knees, and has been coping for a long time without a lot of medication. The slow pace of her knee OA is typical. Several studies have found that, when knee X-rays are repeated after 10 years, only about a third show any impor-tant worsening.

Catherine is not so typical in that her knee OA involves mostly the lateral compartment (outer half), giving her 'knock-knees'. This happens in about a quarter of all patients with knee OA. Other parts of the knee are more commonly affected: the medial compartment (inner half) and the patello-femoral space (between the kneecap, or patella, and the end of the thigh bone, or femur). Some have OA in more than one compartment of the knee. When the inner half of the knee is affected, the resulting deformity is a 'bow-leg'. When OA occurs behind the kneecap (patello-femoral OA) there is often much more muscle weakness, pain and disabil-ity than with the other kinds. Whichever compartment is involved, the process is usually symmetrical, so you don't see a 'knock-knee' on one side and a 'bow-leg' on the other.

Another type of person develops knee OA. These people are much younger, male and have had some sort of knee injury, and often knee surgery.

Ian fits all of these criteria – he's 28, and four years ago he suffered a triple knee injury in a skiing accident. He had arthroscopic surgery to trim the torn cartilage and replace the ligament with 'plastic rope'. Chances are high that over the next 10 to 20 years he's going to start having knee pain and instability, and some typical X-ray changes.

Example 2 – Nodal osteoarthritis of the hands

Here is another example of OA, one that is quite different.

Alice is 45. She runs a small business, selling quilting supplies and giving lessons in quilt-making. She's worried. Her hands, which she considers her livelihood, have been giving her increasing difficulty over the past two years. The problem started soon after the menopause.

'I don't know what I'll do if I become crippled,' she tells me. 'I have a cousin with rheumatoid arthritis. Her fingers are so twisted that she can barely hold a cup of tea without using both hands. Is there anything I can do so that doesn't happen to me?'

I look at her hands, and in particular at the knuckles – the MCP joints at the base of each finger, the middle PIP joints and the end (DIP) joints. The MCP joints look normal to me, but four of the DIPs on each hand and the index finger PIP joint on her right hand are enlarged and lumpy. Several of the DIP joints look red as well.

'I didn't pay much attention at first. It started in my right index finger, at the end. It got very swollen and red, and if I banged it, it hurt. I kept hoping it would go away, and after a couple of months it did. But it left the knuckle stiff and bumpy. Then it spread to another knuckle, and the same thing happened. Now two more have started. They ache constantly, and sting if I hit them, and my fingers are all getting stiff. In the morning it takes about 20 minutes to get them loosened up. I've been taking coated aspirin, and that helps some.'

I ask a few more questions. She is right-handed, and the problem seems to be worse in that hand. She has no symptoms of arthritis except in the hands, and she's in excellent health. She has been asking other members of her family if they've had arthritis. Her mother and two of her three sisters also have 'bumpy' knuckles, but none of them has ever noticed redness or much besides some stiffness in the morning.

Alice has nodal osteoarthritis, probably the most common form of OA, affecting about 75 per cent of women and 50 per cent of men by the age of 70. In middle age, women are affected four times more often than men, and there seems to be an inherited aspect to it. Someone who has it probably has a mother or sisters with it, although inheritance doesn't predict whether it's going to be mild or severe. In women it often comes on at, or just after, the menopause, suggesting a hormonal aspect. Activity also seems to play a role. In right-handed people, more right-hand knuckles are affected, especially in the fingers that are used most.

Many will have local inflammation when the swelling first develops. Redness and marked tenderness usually settle down after several months, leaving the knuckles characteristically 'lumpy' (see Figure 4.1). Individual knuckles are affected at different times. It's not really possible to predict which one will be involved next, or which will be spared. Eventually, no new joints are involved and the hands remain stable thereafter.

The 'lumpiness' is due to new bone being laid down at the margins of the joint. When this lumpiness affects the end (DIP) joints, we speak of *Heberden's nodes*. (William Heberden was an 18th-century physician who was the first person to pay attention to these 'little knobs' [he was also the first person to describe the chest pain we now know as 'angina']. A Frenchman, Charles Bouchard, took second place – he got his name on the middle [PIP] knobs.) Sometimes, when Heberden's nodes are forming, a small cyst over the knuckle develops. If this is punctured, a clear jelly-like material drains out.

Only very rarely are the MCP joints involved; when they are, there may be another kind of arthritis in addition to OA.

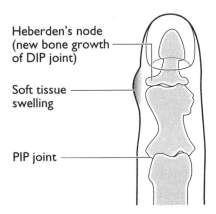

Figure 4.1 Finger osteoarthritis

OA may also occur in the joint at the base of the thumb where it pivots on the wrist (the thumb CMC, or carpometacarpal, joint). This isn't clearly linked to either DIP or knee OA, and it tends to be worse in the non-dominant hand (on the left in a right-handed person). Pain in this joint may be a real problem, especially when the thumb is needed for pinching. A local cortisone injection may help, and sometimes I ask the occupational therapist to fashion a splint to stabilise this joint. Occasionally, I ask a hand surgeon to assess whether surgery would improve the pain and function.

Nodal OA may be quite uncomfortable at times (and without symptoms at others). It may make the fingers look bent, and may make tight gripping difficult. It does not, however, cause the kind of disability that is associated with finger involvement in other kinds of arthritis.

We know that people with nodal OA, like those with lifelong obesity, are more likely to have OA of the knees. However, they do not get arthritis elsewhere with any greater frequency than might be expected by chance. Also, like OA in general, nodal OA is not part of a systemic disease that affects organs such as the heart, lungs and kidneys.

Example 3 – Osteoarthritis of the hip

George is a 65-year-old farmer. He still gets up every morning and is out to the barn before breakfast. His son, though, has taken over most of the running of the farm. That's a pretty good thing, because George's right leg has been bothering him more and more over the past two years. His wife, Mary, comes with him to my office. That turns out to be very helpful, because it's obvious that George tries to play down his problem. She isn't about to let him get away with it, not after waiting so long for this appointment.

'It's my right leg, Doc,' he says. 'I think it's my knee. It's a little stiff when I get out of bed in the morning.' Mary chips in, 'Sometimes he can't even get his sock and shoe on, and I have to do it for him.'

'It's OK as long as I don't push it, but if I'm on my feet much I notice it. The aching does make it hard to get to sleep.'

I'm a little suspicious, as I've been misled before by patients complaining about knee pain when the problem was really in the hip. I ask a few more questions, and I'm glad I did. His pain is mostly in his thigh, in the front of the leg just above the knee. It's in the knee, too. But he also mentions that, if he tries to get into the back seat of his son's car, he gets a pain in the right groin that just about takes his breath away.

His wife confirms that he's never been sick a day in his life. She's certain that neither he nor any other family member has ever had arthritis problems.

My examination confirms my suspicion. The right knee is perfectly normal, but he can barely bend the right hip to 90 degrees, can't roll it inward and can't take it out to the side more than 30 degrees. I'll be very surprised if the X-ray doesn't show that the cartilage is completely gone on the right hip joint.

I tell George and Mary that I'd like to do an X-ray. I also want to make an appointment for him to see an orthopaedic surgeon. I'm not sure he's ready for surgery right now (in fact, I'm pretty sure he's not), but it will be about four months before he can be seen and the first date for elective surgery probably won't be for a year. There's a very good chance he'll be ready by then. Surgery, with replacement of the joint by an artificial one, is almost certain to make a huge difference on his pain and disability. I tell him this, but I also want him to hear it from the surgeon, who also has to tell him about some of the risks involved.

In the meantime, I'm going to arrange for a physiotherapist to see him, show him how to use a cane properly and give him a muscle-strengthening programme.

George has osteoarthritis of the hip. The hip joint is frequently the only one involved in this kind of OA. It's seen about equally in men and women. In a very few cases there's an obvious cause, such as a birth abnormality. Congenital dislocation of the hip is one: an abnormally shallow acetabulum (the cup in the pelvis where the thigh bone fits) allows the hip joint to dislocate and cause damage. Another birth abnormality, one leg being longer than the other, can also be a cause.

Hip OA can occur at any age but most of the people affected are in their 60s and 70s. Some cases are like those of knee OA and go on for a long time with minor symptoms before surgery is necessary. A very few, probably less than 5 per cent, seem to heal on their own. But once people are in enough pain to come to see me, they will usually be more than ready for surgery within two to three years. I usually let the patient define 'ready'. Pain and disability are a far better guide than the X-ray.

George also demonstrates something doctors call 'referred pain'. He feels most of his pain in the thigh and knee area, and not where it belongs – in the groin. Most of the time that a patient comes to me complaining of hip pain, he or she has pain on the outside of the upper thigh or in the buttock. While pain in these areas may be associated with hip problems, it's usually caused by something else.

Example 4 – Osteoarthritis of the spine

Sam is 48 and teaches English. He's a good friend, and so didn't hesitate to call me to give him some information and advice. A week ago he awoke with neck pain that ran down as far as his right shoulder. Now, any attempt to turn his head intensifies it, which makes just about anything he does very difficult. Pain pills help a little, but he's starting to worry that he's taking too many. His family doctor arranged X-rays of his neck. Sam was dismayed to learn that the report was 'extensive degenerative changes involving most of the facet joints, with narrowing of the intervertebral foramina. There is narrowing of C5–6 and 6–7 disc spaces with significant anterior osteophytes at these levels. Advanced OA of the cervical spine.' This sounds serious. Sam wants a translation into something he can understand.

I examine him. There is no suggestion that any of the nerves emerging between the neck vertebrae are being pressed on. His reflexes, his strength and his sensation in both arms are all normal. I look at his X-rays. They don't look like the X-rays of a newborn babe but for someone almost 50 they look pretty good. I have no quarrel with the report but I know two things Sam doesn't. Almost everybody over 40 has changes like this, some better and some worse; and there is absolutely no telling from the X-ray whether the patient has, or ever will have, neck pain.

So I reassure Sam that he will settle down soon. I refer him to a physiotherapist who will probably see him every day until things improve, each time packing his neck in ice and following that with some gentle traction. She'll give him a soft neck collar to wear to bed at night, and offer some advice about pillows. She will not – and I would not – suggest he see a chiropractor because I would worry that neck manipulation might cause serious nerve and blood-vessel damage.

Sam has spinal osteoarthritis. Spinal OA is so common that it's difficult to consider it a disease. Rather, like grey hair, it's something to be expected as we age. The discs between the vertebrae lose some of their water content, shrink and become less bouncy. We lose an inch in height. The facet joints at the back of the vertebrae, which stabilise the spine while still allowing movement, are pushed together. New bone grows in the places where 'mechanical' stresses are high. Most of the time we aren't even aware this has gone on. Sometimes, however, there is local irritation; we experience pain, the supporting muscles go into spasm to keep movement to a minimum, we get more pain and then we call the doctor. Only very rarely is there a serious problem such as nerve pressure, and even more rarely is surgery indicated.

These changes can be seen anywhere in the spine. They are most commonly associated with symptoms in the back (see the section 'Low back pain', later) and, to a lesser extent, in the neck.

So what is osteoarthritis?

Osteoarthritis is defined by the changes that are seen on an X-ray of the joint with symptoms. Compared to a normal joint (see Figure 4.2), the X-ray more or less reveals, depending on the joint and on how long the problem has been going on:

- narrowing of the space between the bones on each side of the joint (the narrowing occurs because cartilage, which doesn't show up on X-ray, has been worn down);

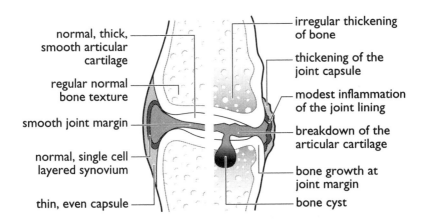

Figure 4.2 Normal versus osteoarthritic synovial joint

- thickening of the bone ends on each side of the joint (bone reacts this way because it has lost the protective 'cap' of cartilage);

- development of cysts in the bone ends (the thicker new bone isn't as elastic as normal bone and, when weight is put on it, tiny fractures occur; fluid from the joint, under pressure, works its way through the cracks into the low-pressure bone, where it expands into cysts);

- growth of bone 'spurs' at the edges of the joint (this is also the body's attempt at healing and strengthening the damaged joint; the Heberden's nodes of nodal OA are really bone spurs of this type).

By this definition, OA can be found in virtually everyone over 50, and in many much younger people. These changes – I cannot emphasise this too strongly – cause symptoms or problems in very few of the people who have them.

Some changes in the joint don't show up on X-ray:

- the cartilage is cracked with tiny fissures, or pitted with ulcerations;

- the lining of the joint is thickened and may be mildly inflamed;

- the capsule that surrounds the joint has become thickened;

- the fluid that lubricates the joint has increased in volume, is often more watery and contains debris from deteriorating cartilage and some inflammatory white blood cells.

These changes will occur in any joint once the cartilage deteriorates. All four common types of OA have really only one thing in common – the cartilage has deteriorated.

How cartilage deteriorates

Cartilage is a tough, spongy, whitish layer that covers bone ends where they meet in a joint. It's living tissue that grows, breaks down and repairs itself. The first step in the development of OA occurs when the repair process no longer matches the rate of breakdown. Sometimes this happens because the cartilage itself is abnormal, such as in chondrocalcinosis. In most cases, though, cartilage breakdown occurs because abnormal stresses, either mechanical or chemical, are brought to bear on normal cartilage.

A brief lesson on cartilage

Cartilage has no blood supply and no nerves; it gets its nutrition and oxygen from joint fluid. Its only cells are chondrocytes, which make the cartilage that surrounds them.

Cartilage consists of two main materials: collagen and proteoglycans (PGs). The collagen forms a tight mesh of tough 'cables' that anchor the whole cartilage structure to the underlying bone. This mesh traps molecules of proteoglycan. Proteoglycans have two very curious properties – they attract water molecules and, like similar poles of two magnets, repel other proteoglycan molecules. Because they sop up as many water molecules as they can, while repelling all other PG molecules trapped in the collagen mesh, about 80 per cent of cartilage is trapped water.

This results in a structure much like one of those 'bubbles' that cover some tennis courts in the winter. The collagen mesh is the fabric of the bubble, and trapped water molecules are the air that is constantly being blown in.

If you can imagine bouncing up and down on a tennis bubble, you can imagine what happens when you take a step. The cartilage covering the bone ends in the knee (hip, ankle, etc.) is compressed as body-weight pressure squeezes some of the trapped water out onto the surface of the cartilage. This does two things. It provides a thin film of liquid for the two cartilage surfaces to slip and glide on as they move against each other. It also squeezes out waste products, including carbon dioxide, from the cartilage. When the body weight is shifted back to the other leg, the cartilage springs back to its original shape and water is sucked back in by the proteoglycans along with oxygen and nutrients such as glucose. So cartilage doesn't need blood vessels for nutrition and oxygen, or to get rid of wastes, as long as it's exercised regularly.

Who gets osteoarthritis?

At one time, OA was simply thought of as a disease of old age. We know better now. Although it's true that the number of people with OA increases with increasing age, many people – even in their 80s – have perfectly normal hips, knees and hands. And we see examples of OA in young and middle-aged adults, without any obvious reason. This has stimulated research into cartilage, in an attempt to determine if many of these people are born with, or develop, cartilage abnormalities that make them more susceptible to deterioration. We also know that knee OA is more likely in people who have (or have a history of) nodal OA.

The treatment of osteoarthritis

There is no single way to treat OA. Age and activity level, the joint or joints involved, the nature of symptoms – all these have to be considered, and the picture can change with time. That's why it's important to keep in touch with a knowledgeable doctor.

Once the diagnosis has been made, it's important for the person to get the message that OA is not simply a disease of 'getting old', that things will not inevitably go downhill and that there's a great deal that he or she can do. Occupational therapists and physiotherapists are often the best source of this message, and should be turned to at least as often as the doctor if things aren't going well.

Prevention

There is now strong evidence of significant risk factors for OA of the knees. It is strong enough that attempting to reduce these risks make sense:

- Obesity in young women (but not men) is a strong predictor for later knee OA. Those who successfully lose weight (one study suggested that as little as 5.4 kg, or 12 pounds, was important) can reduce their risk by over 50 per cent.

- Jobs involving climbing more than ten flights of stairs daily, or repeated kneeling, increase the risk of knee OA threefold, and jobs involving repeated squatting increase the risk more than sixfold.

- Recreational knee injuries that result in cartilage tears or serious ligament strains increase the risk of knee OA at least threefold.

Repeated attempts to link jogging to later hip or knee OA have failed; in fact, there are now good studies demonstrating the reverse. One US study followed 450 middle-aged runners for 12 years, and found that they had fewer joint symptoms, disabilities and medical problems in general than members of a similar group who did not jog regularly. The study continued to follow them a further eight years, into their 60s, and the gap widened. The runners had a third the disabilities of those who didn't jog regularly. However, the same cannot be said for athletes at the elite or professional level – even in non-contact sports such as track and field.

Physiotherapy

People with OA are significantly less fit generally but this can be changed. Restoring fitness in patients with knee OA, by something as simple as supervised indoor walking, has improved both function and pain significantly. At the same time, the need for medication is reduced.

Localised therapeutic exercise is also a potent weapon in dealing with OA, particularly of the knee and hip. Muscles weakened by lack of use are strengthened, and these provide support and protection to the joints, which are vulnerable to further injury in the course of normal daily activities. Pain is reduced. In addition, attention to the hip and knee, including posture correction, can reduce the likelihood of back pain due to awkward standing and walking.

An experienced physiotherapist can analyse the problem and prescribe the right exercise routine, and then reassess the problem at a later date, making any necessary adjustments. Physiotherapy can also help to restore a normal range of movement, which is often lost when a joint becomes painful and is used sparingly. There are many settings for therapeutic exercise: a swimming pool, with the water at a comfortable temperature, is a good place to start. Ice packs or hot packs may help somewhat in reducing discomfort but there is little benefit from most of the electrically powered gadgets that are often used (TENS, or transcutaneous electrical nerve stimulation, and acupuncture also fit into this category of doubtful treatments). Not least of all, a good physiotherapist can help the patient have a realistic perspective on the problem.

Once learned, the exercise programme must be continued daily. This requires commitment; the motivation and the effort must come from the individual. Skipping sessions inevitably results in poor outcome.

Occupational therapy

Occupational therapists (OTs) deal with practicalities. They are skilled in assessing the effect of home and workplace activities on the problem, and vice versa. They can then suggest different ways of doing the job, or tools that will make it easier. Something as simple as having a raised toilet seat can make a huge difference to someone with knee OA. A cane, fitted correctly and used properly, can reduce the load on the hip by as much as 30 per cent.

Occupational therapists are also specialists in providing lightweight splints to support injured joints. Their ability to analyse footwear needs, and to modify shoes with lifts and insole supports, is particularly helpful in OA of the knee, hip and back. For example, placing a soft wedge support into each shoe, under the inner side of the foot, might make a great difference to our 'knock-kneed' first patient, Catherine. The popularity of trainers and walking shoes these days makes the job easier. These provide excellent support and cushioning, at a reasonable price, and can easily be modified for the individual patient.

Drug therapy

No drug can reverse or halt the disease process in OA, but drugs can help relieve symptoms.

For many years, doctors have tended to rely on NSAIDs as first-line treatment of OA. Examples include aspirin, ibuprofen, ketoprofen and indometacin. Although these drugs reduce inflammation and to some extent reduce pain, the results have been at best disappointing and at worst disastrous. Most people with symptoms from OA are over 60, the age group most likely to have adverse effects from NSAIDs. Worsening of pre-existing kidney and heart conditions is common. Ulcers of the stomach or bowel often strike without warning.

Not only do NSAIDs not protect the joint from further damage but there's also some evidence that the reverse may be true. Indometacin seems to accelerate hip OA deterioration, and the same may be true with other drugs.

Recommendations for OA treatment drawn up by the European League Against Rheumatism (EULAR) focus on the use of analgesics (pain-killers) – specifically, *paracetamol*. For many people, regular doses – such as 500 milligrams four times a day, building up if needed to 1,000 milligrams four times a day – are equal, or superior, to NSAIDs. Caution is needed if someone is also taking a blood-thinner, because paracetamol can enhance the effect of warfarin. Paracetamol is also a poison – accidental overdose is the most common cause of liver failure in the USA.

Guidelines for safe paracetamol use include:

- Limit intake to a maximum of 4,000 milligrams a day.

- Avoid any other medicines (such as cold and sinus remedies) containing paracetamol.

- Limit alcohol intake to less than three drinks a day

Paracetamol with codeine can be used if plain paracetamol doesn't work, but if much is required, or even stronger pain-killers are needed, surgery should be considered.

Cortisone-like drugs (such as prednisone) taken by mouth have no place in the treatment of OA. Many times, though, there seems to be a significant amount of inflammation in an OA joint, and I don't hesitate to inject it with a long-acting form of cortisone. This is particularly true of the knee, where repeated injections over time may be quite effective and – despite what seems to be a common belief to the contrary – safe. There is no 'limit' on the number of times a knee can be injected – I will stop if it no longer seems to give at least a few months of relief. I have also seen very good (if temporary) results from injections at the base of the thumb and – under X-ray guidance – into the hip joint.

A variety of other approaches, depending on the particular form of OA, may be tried. In knee OA, injections of a substance called *hyaluronan* have been advocated for the relief of pain. Despite being widely promoted and used, this treatment has yet to convince me of its value. The series of three injections is expensive and even its enthusiasts don't claim much more than six months of benefit.

Many of my patients are taking *glucosamine*, often in combination with *chondroitin*. Theoretically this chemical provides the raw material to build new joint cartilage. Research results on this are contradictory but a well-designed study, published in *The Lancet* in 2001, concluded that glucosamine use reduced pain and retarded knee cartilage breakdown when taken regularly over a three-year period. Whether it can help OA elsewhere – there is one report of improvement in the back pain of spinal OA – and whether the addition of chondroitin makes a difference remains to be seen. I tell my patients that glucosamine is safe to try, and a three-month trial is worthwhile. Unfortunately, I'm not sure all my patients are getting what the package label claims – unlike the EU, where it is a prescription drug of specified potency, glucosamine is a 'nutritional supplement' in North America and not all brands are the same.

A number of drugs are applied as creams or lotions over painful joints. The theory is that they are absorbed through the skin and work their way into the region of the damaged joint. I don't have much experience with this, but from what I read these may have a limited role in helping deal with local OA pain. Many contain NSAIDs, and this way of using them does avoid the risks of taking them by mouth.

Another drug, *capsaicin*, a derivative of chili peppers, may be helpful when applied locally, if nodal or knee OA is very painful. Capsaicin is absorbed through the skin and depletes the nerve ends of 'substance P'. Substance P is a chemical pain messenger, and, if it's not in the nerve endings, pain sensation is reduced. Capsaicin has to be applied several times a day, however, which is a disadvantage. Nevertheless, a recent well-designed study found that a four-times-daily application of capsaicin did make a difference in pain control.

In the future, expect to hear of drugs that retard cartilage breakdown and promote cartilage repair. These may influence outcome profoundly by acting before deterioration becomes obvious on X-ray.

Surgery

Pain, especially night pain, is the main reason for considering surgery; a significant loss of function is the other. Because surgery can fail, at the time or later, it should never be done unless both patient and surgeon are convinced of its necessity. However, delaying too long may jeopardise the outcome. A patient who hasn't walked for two years because of knee OA is not likely to walk again, ever, even with new metal and plastic knees.

There are a number of surgical possibilities, and these vary with the joint involved.

The arthroscope, a small-diameter flexible tube that can penetrate the skin and enter a joint, contains both an optical system for inspecting the joint and the tools needed for microsurgery. It was not uncommon for me to refer a patient to an orthopaedic surgeon for arthroscopic debridement (trimming bits of rough cartilage) and lavage (washout of the joint) – until a recent well-designed study convinced me otherwise. Patients subjected to 'sham' arthroscopic surgery did every bit as well as those who got the real thing.

Tibial osteotomy involves cutting into, 'breaking' and resetting the shinbone (tibia) in cases of knee OA where the surgeon wants to postpone putting in a new artificial joint. This is sometimes done in younger people who have OA of only one side, or compartment, of the knee. By 'bending' the tibia in the right direction, weight can be shifted from the 'sick' side of the knee to the normal side.

Joint fusion, operating to fix the joint in one position permanently, is seldom a good choice in large joints such as knees and hips. It may, however, be an excellent choice in people with severe wrist or elbow pain, or where an important joint, such as a thumb MCP, is unstable.

Total hip replacement – *arthroplasty* – is now almost always successful, and total knee replacement is not far behind. There are still failures, almost always after some time – metal and plastic can break down, cement and bone can give way – but patients should expect at least 10–15 years before such problems arise. Complications such as infection and phlebitis (post-operative blood clotting in leg veins) are still major concerns. Arthroplasty is done only after serious consideration of the alternatives.

Total arthroplasty for other joints remains in the developmental stage; shoulders and elbows are done occasionally but usually only for severe pain and then with the knowledge that function may be no better. The next few years will probably bring new materials and new surgical techniques that will result in the same gratifying results as those we see in hips and knees.

Low back pain

Dave is 50 and an advertising agency executive. He is addicted to running. There are few mornings when he doesn't get in at least an hour, and some days he 'doubles' at noon as well. Six months ago, he put in a long run – a little over two hours – on a Sunday morning. The next day, he became aware of a stiffness across the small of his back. Several hours later he felt sharp pain in that area when he bent over. For the next two weeks he was in misery. Any attempt at forward bending, such as to tie up his shoes, set off a painful spasm. Sleep was safe unless he was on his stomach; then, if he tried to roll over, he would awaken with muscle spasms. He gamely tried to keep running but it was just too painful. After ten days of rest, the pain was still there, but better. At this point, frustrated, he went to see a chiropractor. X-rays showed narrowing of the disc spaces between the lowest three vertebrae in his back. This, it was explained, required adjustment three times weekly. By the second treatment, Dave's pain was significantly better, and in a week he was back to his usual routine. The chiropractor advised monthly manipulation, indefinitely, to prevent a recurrence, but Dave didn't have the time. He was too busy running. He seems to be cured of his pain.

Acute low back pain is a symptom, not a disease.

The lower back is referred to by doctors as the lumbar spine, or the lumbosacral region. Pain there can arise from many sources. It can come from vertebral bone, from the joints or the intervertebral discs that allow one vertebra to move on another, from the ligaments and muscles that tie them together, from the nerves that emerge from the spinal cord or from the spinal cord itself. Pain can also come from nearby structures, particularly those at the back of the abdomen (pancreas, kidney, gut, large blood vessels). Figure 4.3 is a side view of the spine.

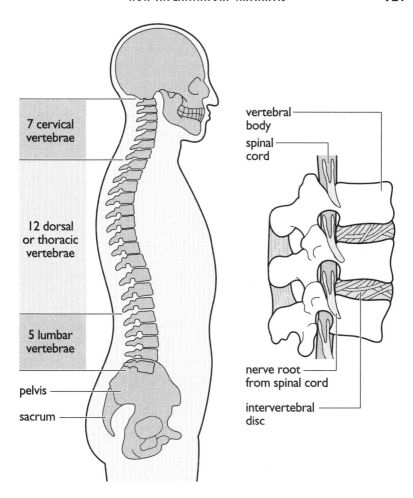

Figure 4.3 The spine

By far the most common back pain is the one Dave experienced. Attempts to pinpoint the source of this type of pain have been failures. Doctors assume that it comes from some localised area of injury in the spine. In most cases it's briefly painful and then heals. This type of pain is often spoken of as 'mechanical low back pain' to distinguish it from inflammatory back pain. It may be sharp or dull, persistent or intermittent. It's felt in the 'hollow' of the back – at waist level, just above the buttocks – but may also spread into one or both buttocks, and occasionally into the back of the thigh.

Pain can develop suddenly, or come on gradually over several days. It may be provoked by an innocent movement, such as bending over, twisting or lifting. It may have no apparent cause. Certain movements may make it quite severe – bending forward or arching backward. Coughing, sneezing or other straining movements may make it worse, as may prolonged sitting in a car. Rest usually helps a lot.

Some generalisations can be made:

- low back pain is common (in any year 10–15 per cent of adults will have an attack);

- most low back pain gets better;

- the cause of most low back pain is unknown.

A sudden attack of low back pain severe enough to interfere with daily life will be experienced, sooner or later, by 80 per cent of us. And, having had one attack, a third will have another within the following three years. People with back pain make up half of all patients who go to family doctors with 'arthritis'.

The likelihood of back pain increases with age, but most patients are men in their 30s, 40s and 50s. A job that involves repeated bending, lifting and twisting often seems to be the cause, although a desk job doesn't provide immunity. Bouncing and vibration, as on a tractor seat or the seat of a long-distance lorry, are also risk factors. Obesity and smoking seem to increase the risk as well.

Low back pain attacks get better spontaneously. Half are gone within one week, and almost all within eight weeks, no matter what is done; a cynic might say this is why chiropractic manipulation seems to be so helpful. Unfortunately, in 5–10 per cent of cases it persists longer than two months. These patients become very frustrated with their pain, and give low back pain its bad reputation. The case of Antonio, described shortly, is a good example: all too often, patients like him are repeatedly, fruitlessly and expensively investigated. If they are really unlucky, they are also subjected to surgery in a vain attempt at a cure.

The truth is that we can't explain most episodes of back pain. There are many potential causes and a large number of possible sources, but attempts to direct treatment to specific back structures generally end in failure. I think most back pain comes from non-bony tissues, including the muscles that support and protect the spinal column.

Despite this, each new back-pain patient I see requires a careful history and examination. I must make sure that the symptom is indeed the common or garden variety of mechanical low back pain (like Dave's), and not back pain that we can, and must, do something about.

Joanne is 34, an associate professor in the faculty of social science and a mother of two very active pre-schoolers. Her back pain began like Dave's, with a gradual onset of deep, aching discomfort across the hollow low in the back. Unlike Dave, however, she experienced more and more pain with each day. Soon the pain was constant. Sitting, particularly in a car, resulted in terrible intensification of pain; lying in bed required careful positioning with pillows. Sleep was constantly interrupted. After a week, sudden movement, coughing and the straining associated with bowel movements (the pain-killers she was taking had given her severe constipation) caused pain to shoot down her right leg and into her foot. The outside of her right foot became numb.

I saw her after this had been going on for three weeks. I attempted to raise her right leg from the examining table but at 30 degrees the pain, quickly moving up the leg to her back, prevented going any further. I asked her to stand on one foot and raise her heel clear of the floor. She could do this on the left foot but not on the right. She was numb on the outer third of the top of her foot. When I struck the back of her ankle with my reflex hammer the usual reaction of calf muscle contraction just didn't happen.

All this – the numbness, the weakness, the loss of the ankle reflex – added up to pressure on a nerve root, and from my examination I was pretty sure this was coming from the very lowest spinal disc space. X-rays of the back were normal, but CT scanning confirmed my suspicion – a protrusion of the disc was causing direct pressure on the nerve root. Here, the clear-cut physical examination findings exactly matched the CT image. Occasions when back surgery can actually be helpful are uncommon but this was one of them. Joanne had her surgery and today, three years later, the only evidence that she ever had a problem is the continued absence of the ankle reflex.

Acute low back pain with nerve root pressure is uncommon (it occurs in only about 1 per cent of people with low back pain), but when it happens, and the pain seems to shoot below the knee in one or both legs, it is called 'sciatica'. This type of pain is usually sharper, and is often made worse by straining movements. It can be associated with tingling, numbness and even weakness in the lower leg and foot. Sometimes the person loses control over bladder or bowel emptying (this is very rare, but it's a surgical emergency).

Joanne's case illustrates the importance of a careful physical examination. If testing raises the possibility that there might be pressure on a nerve, further studies – nowadays CT or MRI scanning – are usually done. Only if the suspicion is confirmed should surgery be considered as an alternative to watchful waiting.

Antonio is 49, and had been an automobile plant production-line supervisor. He hadn't worked for two years, however, and was sent to me for a second opinion. Nine years earlier he'd begun experiencing episodes of intermittent low back pain. These always cleared up in a matter of weeks. Two years ago he again developed pain in the small of his back, which radiated down the back of his upper left thigh. Unfortunately, this time it failed to get better. Indometacin hadn't helped, and physiotherapy, in his case mostly local application of heat and ultrasound, did nothing. The pain was considerably better when he lay flat, so he spent many hours each day stretched out on the rug at home. Sitting longer than 30 minutes was intolerable, and standing more than 15 minutes had the same effect. He denied feeling numbness and tingling in his legs.

Examination showed a stocky and slightly overweight middle-aged man who moved very gingerly. While sitting, he constantly shifted his weight from buttock to buttock. When I asked him to stand and bend forward he did so, slowly, but was unable to arch backward in the standing position. His muscle strength was excellent. He could walk easily on his heels and his toes. The sensation and reflexes in his legs were normal. Plain X-rays of his back showed some minor narrowing of the space between lumbar vertebrae 4 and 5 (L4–5 intervertebral space).

Subsequently Antonio was instructed in a programme of flexion exercises, and purchased a portable back support. He has unfortunately not returned to work and is on long-term disability, with no material change in his symptoms.

Chronic low back pain, long-term and persisting despite all interventions, represents only a small fraction of back pain but constitutes the central problem of back pain in society today. It consumes enormous resources. It has been estimated by BackCare that the healthcare and physiotherapy costs of back pain in the UK amount to about £290 million annually). There are also indirect costs arising from absence from work and disability.

We have very little insight into the causes of this problem. Investigations, even such special ones as MRI and CT scanning, can't distinguish people with chronic low back pain from those with episodic back pain or even from many who have never had any trouble with their backs. Anti-inflammatory drugs aren't helpful, and surgery invariably either does nothing or makes things worse.

There are a few things we have learned about patients like Antonio. The longer they are off work, the less likely they are ever to return. After two years, the chances are less than 5 per cent (see Figure 4.4).

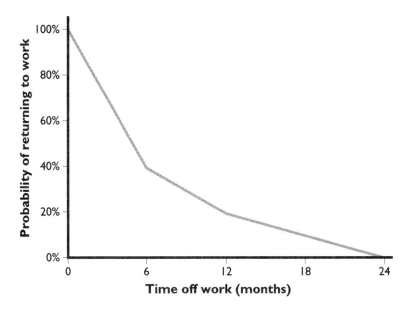

Figure 4.4 Recovery from work-related low back pain. The probability of never returning to work increases with time off work after the injury.
(Adapted from Frymoyer and Cats-Baril, 1991.)

Edith is 74, a retired librarian who lives with her Labrador retriever in a small country cottage five miles from town. She looks much younger than her years, and hasn't an extra ounce of fat on her body, in part because of her daily rambles across the fields and through the wooded area at the back of her property. In the past six months, however, her walking has been severely curtailed by discomfort in the right buttock and leg. She describes it as a cross between pain and weakness. It disappears when she's sitting or lying but comes on with walking. Initially present only on long walks, it has become increasingly easily provoked. Now, just about the time she makes it to the end of the lane to her mailbox, the pain has built to such a pitch that she must sit down. Ten minutes later she can walk again but she barely makes it home. The same thing happens when she stands to wash dishes at the sink. She has discovered she can make it around the supermarket by leaning forward with both arms on the shopping cart.

My examination turns up very little except that she has limited spinal movement and her ankle reflexes can't be detected (something very common in older people). I can easily feel the blood vessels pulse at her ankles and on the tops of her feet.

Edith has lumbar spinal stenosis – a narrowing of the spinal canal most commonly caused by a combination of backward bulging of the disc, bony overgrowth due to osteoarthritis and thickening of one of the spinal ligaments. The narrowing is aggravated by upright posture, which causes a slight degree of extension (backward bending) in the lower spine, which narrows the spinal dimensions even more. (Leaning forward on the shopping cart tends to flatten out the lumbar spine and 'open up' the spinal canal.) Symptoms of spinal stenosis – leg and calf pain with walking – can be mistaken for 'intermittent claudication'. This is a very similar, and common, pain syndrome caused by narrowing of one or more large arteries in the legs. Her normal foot pulses and the abnormal CT scan of her lower spine helped make up my mind. Like so many other tests, the CT scan is useful only if it confirms the history and physical findings; up to 25 per cent of normal people show spinal narrowing on a CT scan but never have a symptom of spinal stenosis.

Many people with spinal stenosis put up with the limitations imposed by the pain and weakness, and some show definite improvement with time. Physiotherapy to strengthen the abdominal muscles and improve spinal posture can help. But some patients, and Edith is one of them, are unwilling to accept their status quo. Edith chose surgery to open up the spinal canal, although she was aware that about a quarter of those who choose surgery end up unhappy with the result.

What else can cause back pain?

Inflammation of the back
Inflammation of the back is nowhere as common as mechanical low back pain. For this reason it's often overlooked – which it shouldn't be because, like inflammatory pain elsewhere, it has a characteristic pattern. More important, it can be treated.

It's worse with rest, and often awakens the person at night. Back stiffness is particularly bad on first arising, and gets much better with physical activity. In contrast, mechanical back pain is almost always better with bed rest and worsens with activity.

The most common type of inflammatory back pain is ankylosing spondylitis. Closely related is the spinal involvement in seronegative arthritis. Back pain may also be part of the picture in polymyalgia rheumatica in older patients. All of these have been covered in Chapter 2.

Nerve root and spinal cord pressure
These are usually signalled by sciatica. Pain is felt not only in the low back region: it spills over into the leg, extends below the knee and may be felt as far as the foot. As in the case of Joanne, the most common cause is a bulging (herniated) intervertebral disc. However, there may be more sinister causes. Cancer involving the spine, benign tumours of the spinal canal or infectious abscesses of the spinal canal are all possible causes. Severe, unrelenting back pain that is continuous both day and night is often the clue to one of these.

Problems in the spinal column itself
These problems include those just mentioned: cancer and infection of either the body of a vertebra or the disc between the vertebrae. The most common cause, however, is a fracture of a vertebral body, and this is almost always due to osteoporosis.

Osteoporosis is the process where bone simply loses its bulk. Bone calcium and the scaffolding on which it's laid down become eroded. When looked at under the microscope, the bone looks moth-eaten instead of being thick and solid.

The typical patient is a post-menopausal woman. Without warning, she develops sudden severe pain in her spine, anywhere from just below the shoulder blades to the lower back. It hurts to move, to cough, to do anything but be very still. Narcotic drugs may be necessary. An X-ray usually confirms the fracture (the vertebral body looks squashed down from its usual square shape into a wedge). The patient gets better, but slowly. By the end of two to three months the pain is gone but the woman may be just a little bit shorter than she was before.

Pain referred to the back from elsewhere

Such pain, usually from within the abdomen, isn't terribly common. Disease of the pancreas, the stomach and duodenum, the kidneys, and the main abdominal artery (the aorta) can all appear as pain in the back.

How should back pain be investigated?

The most important part of the investigation of low back pain is a careful history and physical examination. It's only when things don't make sense, or don't behave as they should, that more is needed. Then the problem is what to choose.

A complete blood count (CBC) and sedimentation rate, two simple blood tests, may be very helpful, especially if inflammation, infection or cancer is on the list of possibilities.

X-rays of the back – reported to make up 5 per cent of all X-rays taken in NHS hospitals – are almost always a waste of money. Furthermore, they may be counter-productive. A recent experiment conducted in general practices in the Nottingham region showed that back pain patients who were X-rayed, compared with those who were not X-rayed, were similar in all respects except for a tendency to have their pain last longer and affect them more severely. They tended to visit their doctors more – and to be more satisfied with their care – than the group who weren't X-rayed! I reserve X-rays for patients in whom the question of fracture, cancer, infection, inflammatory arthritis or nerve damage has been raised. That works out to far less than 10 per cent of patients with back pain.

Other ways to look at the back include CT (or CAT – computed axial tomography) scanning, MRI (magnetic resonance imaging) or radionuclide bone scanning. They are all, in their individual ways, better at 'seeing' spinal structures than plain X-rays. They are also much more expensive and much less freely available. I order them only if I feel that the patient's back pain is different, particularly if I'm considering one of the more unusual causes or if I'm thinking that surgery may be required.

Back pain – what doesn't work

- Surgery (except in specific cases)

- Bed rest

- Traction

- TENS (transcutaneous electrical nerve stimulation)

- Back injections (except for sciatica)

- Back education classes (to prevent work-related injury)

- Muscle relaxants

- Special corsets and belts

A note of caution, however. A study reported in the *New England Journal of Medicine* examined MRI testing in almost 100 people with no symptoms of back pain. Half of these patients showed 'disc bulging' and a quarter showed 'disc herniation'. That normal people have 'abnormal' results of this nature has been suspected for a long time. Similar findings have arisen from studies of CT scans. The lesson is clear: abnormalities found by CT or MRI testing are important only if they fit the patient's symptoms and findings on examination. To operate on the basis of the imaging test alone is to ensure a failure of surgery.

How should back pain be treated?

Obviously the answer varies with the cause, but here I intend to
focus on mechanical low back pain of recent onset. Traditionally,
treatment has been a choice between the surgical option and the
'conservative' option.

The surgical option

Back in the late 1930s, Drs Mixter and Barr popularised the idea
that low back pain was caused by herniation (bulging due to
weakening of the outer fibres) of the intervertebral disc. As a
result, for 40 years patients with low back pain were operated on,
often repeatedly, in an attempt to reduce the disc herniation or to
fuse the vertebrae together, or both. Only in the last decade have
we come to realise how ineffective and harmful this usually was.
Those few people with clear-cut nerve pressure were helped
enormously. But many others, those whose pain we still can't
explain, experienced only continued, if not worsened, pain and
disability.

If there is definite nerve root pressure, surgical relief of that
pressure is usually extremely helpful. But even in these cases,
surgery is not always the only way to improvement. I have had
patients who refused surgery and got better. As MRI studies
have shown that disc bulges often resolve on their own, this is not
surprising.

My current practice is to recommend surgery only if:

- the patient's symptoms and my examination point to nerve
  pressure, *and*

- the CT or MRI agrees with my findings, *and*

- the pain continues to be disabling despite the passage of
  time,

or

- I find evidence that nerve damage is getting worse,

or

- the patient has symptoms of loss of bladder or bowel
  control.

The 'conservative' option

Bed rest, usually for at least two weeks, was the rule 25 years ago, but now we recommend either no rest in bed or rest for only a brief period – preferably just a day or two, until the acute pain passes. Then we try to get the patient moving again. But a number of more specific treatments are also available.

Various *back injections* have been used. The most effective involves injecting the lumbar epidural space (the space between the covering of the spinal cord and the bone of the spinal canal) with a mixture of corticosteroid and long-acting local anaesthetic. This is done to relieve very severe pain, particularly if there is sciatica. It may be necessary to repeat injections over several weeks, but the relief provided can be considerable.

Anti-inflammatory drugs and pain-killers may be very useful, particularly in pain of recent onset. They may allow the patient to resume normal activity more quickly. Because there is generally little or no inflammation in the usual type of back pain, anti-inflammatories, if they do help, usually do so because they also have pain-killing properties. Some doctors also prescribe muscle relaxants, but they have never been proved effective.

Various appliances are also available – from the infrared, ultrasound, shortwave diathermy and interferential machines in physiotherapy departments, to corsets and back braces, and the more recent portable TENS (transcutaneous electrical nerve stimulation) units. The best that can be said of these is that they do no harm – the worst that their use wastes a great deal of time and money. They should never be used – as they are too often – as the sole treatment.

Chiropractic manipulation may be worth a try, at least if the back pain is of recent onset and is not going away. A British study comparing chiropractic and traditional physiotherapy for recent-onset back pain found that patients treated by chiropractors felt better faster.

An American study compared the outcomes of acute low back pain patients treated by family doctors, orthopaedic surgeons and chiropractors. There was no difference in outcome – recovery of function was rapid in almost all patients – but chiropractic treatment was associated with both higher costs and greater patient satisfaction with the treatment.

Current recommendations for treatment of acute low back pain
Because virtually all acute back pain will settle down without any
treatment, most experts in the field now recommend that people
in the early stages – three to four weeks – be given whatever is
needed for pain, reassured of the high probability of complete
recovery and strongly urged to get back to work as quickly as
possible. If early return to work full-time is just too difficult, a
return on a part-time basis should be sought.

Experts now agree that someone who has been off work
between four and twelve weeks is an entirely different problem.
He or she is in real danger of long-term difficulties, as measured
by a successful return to work.

A first step is a reassessment by the doctor to check for an
uncommon, potentially treatable condition (see 'Red flags' box).
Then the principles of 'intensive work-related case management'
are applied. Absolutely essential is the co-operative collaboration
of the worker and the employer, often with the assistance of a
physiotherapist and an occupational therapist. The focus is on the
job. The specific activity involved is analysed. The specifics of the
job may be modified, or the hours on that task reduced, or the
worker may be involved in a specific work-hardening exercise

'Red flags' calling for immediate medical attention

- Age under 20 or over 55

- Pain in the upper back (between shoulder blades)

- Fever, weight loss, night sweats

- Gradual onset, morning stiffness, improvement with
  movement

- Recent severe injury

- Severe night pain

- Symptoms of nerve damage (loss of muscle strength, feeling,
  bowel, bladder control)

- A history of cancer or corticosteroid treatment

Rules for a healthy back

- Become aerobically fit, and keep it up

- Get rid of belly fat

- Learn a simple routine of back strengthening and flexibility exercise, and do it

- Adopt good work postures, especially for lifting

- Wear comfortable, supportive, cushioned, low-heeled work shoes

---

programme – or a combination of all three. (A work-hardening exercise programme gradually adapts the worker to the physical demands of the job.) In workplaces where programmes such as these are available, time lost from work in the first year may be reduced by up to 50 per cent.

Fibromyalgia (fibrositis)

Mary Jane is a 40-year-old woman who balances managing a household and three active teenagers with her full-time job in the medical records department of our hospital. She looks tired and very worried. I ask her why she has come to see me. Her answer is one I've heard so many times before; I have to remind myself that jumping to conclusions is not an official Olympic event.

'Doctor, I hurt all over.'

I ask her to be more specific, and it soon becomes obvious that her pain is indeed widespread – in her neck, her arms, her back and her legs. It's also clear that she points as much to the muscles as to the joints.

'It's been going on for at least six months. At first I thought it was the flu – everyone else in the family had it – but even after the fever and headache cleared up, my muscles still ached.'

By now I can almost predict her answers to my next questions.

'Am I tired? I wake up tired. I feel so weak some days I don't believe I'm going to make it to bedtime. And I'm not getting a good

night's sleep. The littlest thing seems to wake me up, and my husband says I'm tossing and turning all night. And I'm so stiff in the morning! It takes me hours to get loose.'

Mary Jane has a number of other symptoms I've come to recognise as typical. She has always had problems with migraine but lately the headaches have become much more frequent. She has developed symptoms of irritable bowel syndrome – morning clusters of crampy lower abdominal pain ending in, and temporarily relieved by, a loose, watery bowel movement. She has tried taking a variety of anti-inflammatory medications but they don't work. The worst thing, she says, is that she looks so well. None of her joints is swollen, and her family is beginning to think her problem is in her head.

I examine her – first a quick general physical examination, to make sure there is nothing else, and then a more specific assessment, looking for tenderness at each of the nine pairs of fibromyalgia tender points. As I go over each of these, pressing firmly with my thumb, she pulls away in obvious discomfort. She seems amazed that I know exactly where to touch to bring out her pain.

Fibromyalgia is a syndrome defined by widespread musculo-skeletal pain for at least three months, and abnormal tenderness to pressure on at least 11 of 18 specific points (see Figure 4.5).

In order to meet the definition, pain has to be on both right and left sides of the body, and above and below the waist. The tenderness can be measured by pressing each point with an instrument called a 'dolorimeter' (literally, 'pain meter'). Most commonly, though, each location is checked by firm thumb pressure. A number of nearby 'control' sites are also pressed to make sure that the 'tender points' are truly not normal.

Who gets fibromyalgia?

Whilst the typical patient is a middle-aged woman, slightly over-weight and relatively physically unfit, there are a lot of exceptions. I see teenagers and the elderly, along with the athletic, with fibromyalgia. It is one of the most common diagnoses I make.

Chronic pain, felt throughout the body, is common. Studies in both Britain and the USA have come up with similar figures – about 11 per cent of the adult population 'hurts all over'.

The much more specific form of generalised pain, what we call

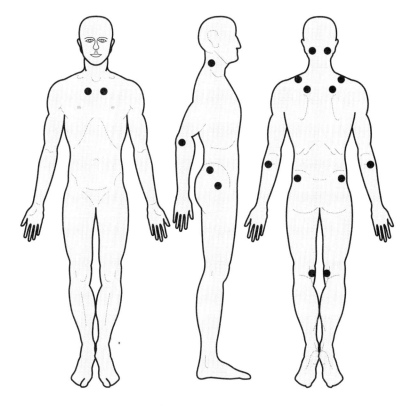

Figure 4.5 The tender points in fibromyalgia

fibromyalgia, is also common, though less so. Probably the best and most meticulously carried out investigation was one done in Canada. It showed that, in a large urban centre, almost 6 per cent of women and 2 per cent of men met the definition. This makes fibromyalgia almost four times as common as rheumatoid arthritis.

What are the characteristics of fibromyalgia?

Muscle pain

Muscle pain is variously described as aching, gnawing or burning, and is the hallmark of fibromyalgia. Mary Jane had difficulty in telling me where, precisely, she hurt; the best she could do was indicate 'all over'. In contrast, my examination pinpointed a large number of locations where she was extremely tender; before I did so, she was unaware of any of them. When I pressed firmly

---

Symptoms of fibromyalgia

- Generalised pain – muscles and joints

- Profound tiredness

- Poor sleep

- Difficulty concentrating and remembering

- Morning stiffness

- Numbness and tingling

---

over other nearby areas, and over her joints, I couldn't get the same reaction.

Fatigue
This is often so severe that the patient believes there's something wrong with the muscle, but the results of extensive muscle testing are always normal and strength is actually quite good. However, the combination of pain and fatigue is deadly. The quality of life has been studied in patients with fibromyalgia and found to be as poor as in patients with chronic obstructive lung disease and insulin-dependent diabetes.

Disturbed sleep
This might be better described as restless sleep, with a tendency to waken easily. This feature may give a clue as to the cause, at least in some people. Drs Hugh Smythe and Harvey Moldofsky, working in Toronto in the 1970s, discovered that patients with fibromyalgia don't sleep the way otherwise normal people do. Sleep patterns can be traced on an EEG (electroencephalogram). Normal people range up and down, from very light sleep (Stage I) to very deep sleep (Stage IV), many times throughout the night. People with fibromyalgia do this as well, but their Stage IV sleep (also called 'slow wave' or restorative sleep) is 'contaminated' with Stage I sleep, as if they never quite fully relax.

Smythe and Moldofsky did something very interesting: they took normal volunteers and hooked them up to EEG machines in the sleep lab, and whenever the volunteers entered Stage IV sleep they were roused slightly – not enough to wake them but enough to disturb their EEG tracings. After several nights of this, the volunteers started waking up tired, stiff and hurting all over.

Morning stiffness

This is one exception to the rule that the symptom is an indicator of inflammation. Testing never detects evidence of inflammation, and symptoms do not respond to treatment for inflammation unless (see below) the fibromyalgia is associated with another type of arthritis. Because morning stiffness is so often combined with fatigue, patients often describe awakening as if they 'had been run over by a lorry'.

Other symptoms

Patients often tell me of numbness and tingling in their hands, though there is never evidence of nerve irritation. They commonly mention that their hands and fingers feel swollen, though there's no swelling that I can detect. Headache and bowel irritability occur in about 50 per cent of cases, and current or past depression and anxiety attacks in about 25 per cent – more often than would be expected by chance. It's not clear whether there's a cause-and-effect relationship with the fibromyalgic pain. What *is* clear is that many people with chronic pain become depressed and anxious, particularly if their doctors can't find anything wrong. They suspect the worst, and when a name can be put to their problem they're delighted.

Look-alikes

Superficially, at least, fibromyalgia may be mistaken for one of any number of rheumatic disorders, including systemic lupus erythematosus, polymyositis (an inflammatory disorder of muscle), polymyalgia rheumatica and even rheumatoid arthritis. Recently I have seen a number of women who were inappropriately labelled as having 'fibromyalgia' who in fact had ankylosing spondylitis.

Hypothyroidism (abnormally low function of the thyroid gland) is a diagnosis I've been fooled on, though, so I make it a habit to order a TSH (Thyroid-Stimulating Hormone) test on everyone who gets a label of 'fibromyalgia'. Unlike fibromyalgia, hypothyroidism is easy, and very satisfying, to treat.

All of these look-alikes have characteristic findings on physical examination, and they usually show definite abnormalities on lab testing. This is quite different from fibromyalgia, where the usual lab tests are normal.

What causes fibromyalgia?

No one knows. Despite its name ('myalgia' means muscle pain and 'fibro-' refers to the tissue surrounding muscle fibres), no specific abnormalities of muscle have been found. There may be many causes.

Trauma, either physical or emotional, is suspected in some cases, simply because of the timing. Some patients' symptoms follow automobile accidents. Some investigators have also raised the possibility of 'microtrauma' as a factor in at least perpetuating the disease. They point out that most patients with fibromyalgia are generally out of shape, and their muscles are more susceptible to small injuries in normal everyday use.

Infection is often suspected as a cause. Commonly, as in Mary Jane's case, the first symptoms appear after a viral-like infection. The virus of infectious mononucleosis has been investigated, and discarded, as a cause. It was suspected in part because it was also a suspect in myalgic encephalomyelitis (ME), Also known as chronic fatigue syndrome (CFS), ME shares the fibromyalgia tender points, sleep disturbances and pain. Fatigue, however, predominates over pain, and patients often have low-grade fever, sore throat and enlarged lymph glands – symptoms that suggest even more strongly an infectious cause.

The link is even more confusing in the case of Lyme disease – an infection caused by a spirochaete passed on to humans by infected ticks (see Chapter 5). One of the symptoms of Lyme disease is arthritis. Unfortunately, Lyme disease is often very hard to diagnose. Symptoms may be confusing, and blood tests aren't reliable. Even in areas where Lyme disease is common, a positive result in a Lyme disease test is four times more likely to be false than true.

Recently, researchers in a Lyme disease clinic in Boston, USA, looked at musculoskeletal symptoms in all the patients they had been following up for a number of years. The average follow-up was almost five years, which was sufficient time to be certain of the diagnosis. Almost half of their patients actually had Lyme disease, either active (23 per cent) or inactive (20 per cent). The rest (57 per cent) had never had Lyme disease. What was startling was that, in both groups, fibromyalgia or myalgic encephalomyelitis was found in over half the patients. This suggests two things: (1) infection with Lyme disease may possibly trigger fibromyalgia, and (2) the symptoms of fibromyalgia may lead to a false diagnosis of Lyme disease. Certainly many people with fibromyalgia have been treated with repeated courses of antibiotics in a futile attempt at curing Lyme disease.

Human immunodeficiency virus (HIV) infection has also been linked to a high frequency of fibromyalgia symptoms.

Other types of arthritis, if they go on long enough, can lead to fibromyalgia on top of the original problem. This is fairly common in rheumatoid arthritis (RA), where shoulder pain often makes sleep very difficult. It makes sense that this might cause the kind of sleep disturbance that Smythe and Moldofsky provoked by slightly rousing volunteers in a sleep lab. When a patient with RA is feeling worse, it's important to recognise whether the problem is fibromyalgia. It's not a good idea to treat the wrong disease.

Abnormalities of pain perception may lie at the root of fibromyalgia, which has been called a 'pain amplification syndrome'. When pain sensation is tested in areas away from the 18 'tender points', people with fibromyalgia are much more sensitive than others. And when patients with fibromyalgia are asked to rate their pain on a scale of 1 to 10, and they are compared to patients with RA, their pain intensity is twice as high. Researchers have found several abnormalities that may explain the heightened sensitivity to pain experienced by people with fibromyalgia. Elevated levels of substance P (a chemical involved in the transmission of pain) have been found in cerebrospinal fluid – the fluid that bathes the brain and spinal cord. They have also documented relative deficiencies of serotonin – another chemical of the nervous system – and subnormal secretion of adrenal gland hormone in response to stress.

There are many – doctors, insurance company executives and even some judges – who don't believe in fibromyalgia. Some see it as a psychiatric disorder, or as conscious malingering. I'm not in that camp. I've seen too many people – emotionally stable, hard-working, with nothing to gain and everything to lose – who have been laid low by fibromyalgia. I believe that, in time, the roots of the problem will be laid bare, and when that happens we will finally have an effective treatment approach.

How is it treated?

Whenever there's a long list of possible treatments for any disorder, you can be sure that none is very good. This is certainly true for fibromyalgia. There is no cure. The goal is to regain control, as much as possible, of a normal life.

Aerobic fitness conditioning

This is used because people with fibromyalgia are generally very unfit – probably as a result of their disease. Improving fitness does result in reduced pain, but it's not known if this effect will hold up in the long run. Most treatment programmes combine fitness conditioning with muscle strengthening and general flexibility exercises. Twenty minutes of each – for a total of one hour – three times a week has been shown to improve the overall level of function. But this regimen must be built up to slowly and painstakingly. Ideally, an experienced physiotherapist should guide the patient along. Postural awareness and correction of bad postural habits can also be taught by the physiotherapist.

Tricyclics

Having recognised that sleep disturbance may be important in fibromyalgia, Smythe and Moldofsky tried a number of drugs that might affect sleep, and settled on amitriptyline. Given in doses much lower than usually used for depression, amitriptyline is very effective in about a third of patients. The majority aren't helped, though. Those who do notice improvement often stop the drug because of unpleasant side effects such as feeling 'zonked out' the next morning, or experiencing constipation or severe dry mouth. Some of those who do carry on find that amitriptyline loses its initial benefit after a while. A number of related compounds, including cyclobenzaprine, give similar, rather disappointing results.

Keeping active
The other main benefit of an exercise programme is to show patients with fibromyalgia that they can exercise and become fit, although their pain and fatigue tell them the opposite. By avoiding physical activity they become less and less fit, so they get caught up in a vicious circle of pain and fatigue leading to inactivity and deconditioning, which results in even more pain and fatigue. It's much like the situation of people with chronic back pain; resting to relieve the pain is exactly the wrong thing to do.

Sleep improvement
Better sleep can be expected with both tricyclic medication and fitness conditioning. Small things, such as changing to a smaller, moulded pillow to support the head and neck in a neutral position, are often surprisingly helpful.

Stress management
Stress is often a major part of the problem, and not just a result of fibromyalgia. It may in fact play a role in its development. Financial worries and abusive marital relationships are surprisingly common among patients. Counselling from an appropriate source may be a key element in coping with fibromyalgia.

Learning about fibromyalgia
It's essential that Mary Jane understand her disease if she is going to keep it from controlling her life. The first step is the diagnosis. She needs to learn that the problem is not 'all in her head', neither will it cripple or kill her. She needs to learn to recognise the various symptoms and not be frightened by them. She must realise that initial attempts at becoming more fit are going to be hard, and possibly even painful, but that in the long run they will pay off.

One of the best ways to learn about fibromyalgia is to link up with a group with the same problem. There are self-help groups devoted to fibromyalgia in many communities. Arthritis Care and the Fibromyalgia Association UK can provide more information.

Analgesics
Pain-killers such as paracetamol may be necessary and helpful, but NSAIDs don't work.

What's the long-term otlook?

This is a hard question to answer, because most patients have been looked at for only short periods. Also, studies have been carried out only in university centres, where the toughest cases are likely to be sent. Those, however, suggest that there is very little change, at least in the short term. At four-year and five-year follow-ups less than a quarter of the patients were better, and most were worse. Those who tended to improve were younger, and had had less overall pain to start with, than those who didn't.

Fibromyalgia seen outside these university centres may be much more benign – that's certainly the case with many other diseases. We know that the vast majority of patients continue to work full time, and those who aren't working should try to return to work. This may require the intensive combined efforts of doctor, physiotherapist and occupational therapist, as well as co-operation from the employer. But the result will be worth the hard and often painful effort.

5
Uncommon Types of Arthritis

Lyme disease

From time to time I see a patient who is very frightened. The patient invariably has the diffuse aches and pains characteristic of fibromyalgia. She or he has heard about Lyme disease, recalls a hiking or camping trip and might even have had a test for Lyme disease, which may or may not have been positive. Some have, in fact, been treated with antibiotics – unsuccessfully.

Why this extraordinary fear? It is probably due to several factors. First of all, Lyme disease is something new and it's infectious. People have heard that it can be serious, and that it can be hard to diagnose. Its symptoms can be confused with symptoms of other conditions. Laboratory tests may not always give clear-cut answers. And there is concern that a delay in treatment might have serious consequences.

Each of these points deserves comment. First, though, I'd like to tell the story of how Lyme disease was discovered.

In November of 1975, Polly Murray made an appointment to see Dr Allen Steere, a Yale University medical scientist. She was an artist and mother of four living in Lyme, Connecticut, and for ten years she had been experiencing mysterious and unexplained symptoms – recurring fatigue, depression, weight loss and low-grade fever. Several times she had attacks of joint pain and swelling. Doctors (she had been examined by many) were unable to explain her symptoms. It had even been suggested that the problem was 'in her head'. But in the months before her appointment with Dr Steere, Mrs Murray's husband and two of her children developed similar symptoms. She asked around, and discovered others in her community who seemed to be affected. By the time she met Dr Steere she had a list of 35 people who had been variously diagnosed with infectious arthritis, systemic lupus erythematosus, rheumatoid arthritis and juvenile rheumatoid arthritis. She was convinced that all had the same condition, and it was due to exposure to some common agent.

Dr Steere believed Mrs Murray, and within several months had identified, in Lyme and in two nearby communities, a total of 39 children and 12 adults who seemed to be suffering from some form of epidemic arthritis. The observation that most cases of arthritis came on in the summer months, and that for many the arthritis had been preceded by a rash resembling one known in Europe to be caused by a tick bite, pointed the search in the right direction. The story unfolded slowly but by 1981 it was evident that Lyme disease:

- is an infection caused by a microscopic organism;

- is passed on to humans by ticks;

- can be successfully treated with antibiotics;

- often starts with a typical skin rash, and can progress to involve the nerves, heart and/or joints.

Even in southern Ontario, where I live (and where possibly only a dozen cases of Lyme disease have been convincingly proved), I am often asked, 'Could I have Lyme disease?'

The risk of exposure to Lyme disease

Lyme disease is caused by an organism that is transmitted to humans by the bite of the *Ixodes* tick. The species of *Ixodes* tick that carries this spirochaete varies with the geographical location, but in New England it is *Ixodes dammini*. Initially this species was near extinction, found only on the island of Nantucket. The appearance of Lyme disease along the eastern seaboard of the USA corresponded to a tick population explosion, undoubtedly helped by its natural hosts, deer and the white-footed mouse. Because humans, mice and deer are increasingly neighbours, particularly as suburbia spreads in the heavily populated coastal corridor from Massachusetts to North Carolina, it's not surprising that occasionally an infected tick bites a human.

Lyme disease and the *Ixodes* tick seem to be spreading further and further each year. Some scientists suspect that, in addition to being carried by deer and mice, the tick may be hitch-hiking on migrating birds.

The seaboard states from Massachusetts to Maryland account for 75 per cent of the more than 10,000 cases reported each year in the USA. Most of the rest are in the northern Midwest (especially Minnesota and Wisconsin) and coastal West (particularly California). However, people with Lyme disease have turned up in every state. Usually this is because they have holidayed in a 'hot' or endemic area. Nevertheless, 'native cases' do occur, even in Canada. Lyme disease is also found throughout most of Europe and northern Asia.

What Lyme arthritis looks like

Soon after the bite, about the time the Lyme skin rash (described below) appears and for up to a month or two afterward, people may experience muscular and joint aches and pains that move about the body without joint swelling.

Lyme arthritis develops, on average, about six months after the initial tick bite. About 50 per cent of those who acquire the infection develop arthritis. Lyme arthritis is quite obvious – the joint involved becomes very swollen and painful. Only one or two joints are affected at a time, and they tend to be large joints, particularly the knees. An affected joint will 'cool off' after days to weeks, but it's common for another (or the same) joint to flare up again later. If the infection is not treated, attacks of single-joint arthritis tend to recur at increasing intervals, each attack just a bit less 'hot' than the last until, some time within two to three years after the initial tick bite, no more attacks occur. Even if the person is adequately treated and the infection cured, it may take several months for the arthritis attacks to wind down.

It's very rare for local inflammation to persist in a joint, and even more uncommon for bone and cartilage damage to develop. In a group of patients diagnosed with Lyme arthritis in the days before antibiotics were known to be effective, only 10 per cent went on to chronic arthritis. In some of these patients, persisting infection may not be the problem. The infection may have triggered the initial arthritis, been eliminated by antibiotics but somehow initiated a process similar to reactive arthritis (discussed in Chapter 2). In such cases, antimalarials and surgical removal of the inflamed joint tissue through an arthroscope have been used successfully.

Lyme arthritis never looks like rheumatoid arthritis, but it can look like one form of childhood arthritis.

As described in Chapter 4, many people with Lyme disease develop symptoms that are classic for fibromyalgia. This poses a problem, because fibromyalgia itself is so common. How can we tell if fibromyalgia symptoms in a given patient are a consequence of Lyme disease? For one thing, we can consider the odds; even where Lyme disease is most commonly seen, fibromyalgia is still far more frequent. We can also take a careful history of exposure and symptoms, and consider the timing of the patient's symptoms when reviewing the results of blood testing. Fibromyalgia symptoms do not mean that the Lyme infection is active, and they do not respond to Lyme disease treatment with antibiotics.

The good news about Lyme disease

The *Ixodes* tick is very small, and may escape detection. But it isn't easy to catch Lyme disease; the tick must remain attached from 36 to 48 hours to pass on the infection. It has been estimated that even in areas where up to 40 per cent of all ticks are infected, only about 1 to 3 per cent of tick bites will result in Lyme disease. With odds like that, a person bitten by a tick in an endemic area and treated with antibiotics 'just in case' is far more likely to get sick from the treatment than from Lyme disease. And people themselves have to be bitten by the tick to be at risk. Although dogs can get Lyme disease, they never pass it on to their owners.

Evidence of Lyme disease elsewhere in the body

In about 5 per cent of cases, arthritis is the first sign of Lyme disease, and sometimes it's the only one. The initial tick bite may not even be remembered – only about a third of patients recall being bitten. A correct diagnosis is therefore easier if other symptoms have been noticed.

The skin rash of Lyme disease, which follows the infected tick bite only 50 to 70 per cent of the time, is called 'erythema chronicum migrans' (ECM). It starts off as a small red bump where the tick has bitten – usually in the area of the armpit, groin or thigh. Over a few days it spreads outward in a rapidly enlarging circle, which may be several inches across. The centre tends to clear as the red spot enlarges, giving the appearance of a 'bull's eye'. Without treatment, the rash clears within several days to weeks. Because it doesn't itch or hurt, if it's tucked away on the back or in the armpit it may not even be noticed.

The heart is affected in 5 to 10 per cent of untreated patients. Symptoms may be absent, or there may be heart rhythm irregularities (palpitations). Dizziness and fainting spells may occur. These symptoms rarely last more than a few weeks.

Nervous system symptoms, which occur in about 10 per cent of Lyme patients, may suggest infection of the brain (meningitis and encephalitis), spinal cord and major nerves in the hands and feet. Headache, neck stiffness, difficulty concentrating and emotional upset can dominate the picture. There can be numbness, pain or weakness in the limbs. A very common symptom is the development of Bell's palsy: the nerve to half the face is affected and that side of the face appears flattened. The corner of the mouth may droop and the smile is distinctly crooked. These symptoms tend to come on two to three months after the skin rash.

Heart and nervous system symptoms get better with treatment, although it may take several months for things to get completely back to normal.

Blood tests for Lyme disease

Blood tests will be negative for the first two to three weeks, and for up to eight weeks in some cases. Blood tests aren't necessary, however, if the evidence is there. If some or all of the clues fit – typical skin rash, memory of a tick bite, presence in an area of known Lyme disease and potential exposure to a tick, and symptoms consistent with Lyme disease – the diagnosis can be made.

Many people test positive for Lyme disease who have never had the disease. About 7 per cent of the general public will have a positive 'ELISA' test (to screen for Lyme exposure), whereas, even in areas where Lyme disease is most frequent, only 1 per cent of tests are true positives. Other infections, mononucleosis, even rheumatoid arthritis, are among the many causes of a positive ELISA. On the other hand, a negative test means just that: the patient does not have, and never has had, Lyme disease, unless the test is done within eight weeks of the bite, or the patient has had antibiotics early in the disease. In the latter case the antibiotics may not have cured the disease, but the test may still be a false negative.

If a patient has a positive ELISA test and the picture is suspicious, a second test – the more specific 'Western blot' test – is done. It too can be negative if done too soon or if the patient has been given antibiotics early on. A positive test isn't the end of it, though. It can give several different answers, all considered 'positive' – but only if the particular answer exactly matches the patient's story.

What's a patient to do?

Where the probability of Lyme disease is high, it should be treated with antibiotics. High probability situations exist where there is a reasonable chance of past exposure to the *Ixodes* tick, where symptoms are consistent with Lyme disease, and where the blood test results fit the picture. Treatment isn't simple. It may involve intravenous antibiotics over three to four weeks.

Where the probability of Lyme disease is low – when a definite diagnosis of the disease has been appropriately treated but the patient continues to be tired, with aches and pains, or when a mistaken diagnosis of Lyme is made based on misinterpreted symptoms and lab tests – the risk of 'pseudo-Lyme' is high. The patient and/or the doctor becomes convinced that Lyme disease is the problem. The result can then be repeated, unnecessary, visits to the doctor, blood tests, courses of antibiotic treatment, side effects of treatment (in up to half the cases), time off work, depression and stress.

Prevention of Lyme disease

The first step is common sense, especially in areas with infected ticks. Avoid woods and brushy areas in the late spring and early summer, when the ticks are most likely to attach. Wear light-coloured long-sleeved garments, and tuck trousers into socks. Inspect yourself or your child carefully, at night before the bath. Any attached ticks should be removed, after cleansing the skin with alcohol, with tweezers or gloved fingers. Don't dig out any mouth parts that remain embedded in the skin – they will be shed in a day or two. And don't forget – a tick has to be attached for more than a day to transmit the disease, and only 1 to 3 per cent of tick bites in areas where Lyme is common actually result in the disease.

There is now a very effective vaccine against Lyme disease but, like all vaccines, it is not guaranteed to be 100 per cent effective. And it only protects against Lyme. Many infected ticks carry other organisms, and the vaccine doesn't prevent the illnesses they cause. So, whilst it may make very good sense to vaccinate – especially children in areas where Lyme disease is common – it's also good sense to keep up measures to prevent and detect tick attachment.

Arthritis in children (JIA)

Arthritis in children is really quite uncommon. It may be a complication of an infection or of cancer, but more commonly the cause is unknown. In the UK, each year there are about 10 cases for every 100,000 children (similar to childhood diabetes).

For many years, the term used in the USA was 'juvenile rheumatoid arthritis' (JRA), whereas in Britain it was known as 'juvenile chronic arthritis' (JCA). Since 1994 there has been an attempt to use the same label on both sides of the Atlantic, and that label is 'juvenile idiopathic arthritis' (JIA). 'Idiopathic' simply means 'the cause is unknown'.

Varieties of childhood arthritis

Arthritis in children usually fits into one of three categories:

- arthritis involving relatively few joints,
- arthritis involving many joints,
- arthritis as part of Still's disease.

Arthritis involving relatively few joints

Doctors call this 'pauciarticular arthritis' ('pauci' means 'few'), and it's the most common of the three. About 55 to 75 per cent of childhood arthritis fits into this category.

Four or fewer joints are affected at any one time, and they tend to be larger joints – a knee, ankle or elbow. Occasionally, small hand joints will also be affected.

Typically, the child is a girl and is less than five years old when the problem begins. Pain may not be very obvious. In fact, up to a quarter of these children don't complain of pain. The first thing noticed may be that the child is limping or is unable to straighten out the leg. The child is usually not otherwise ill. Blood tests for arthritis are negative except for the antinuclear antibody (ANA) test, which is commonly positive and is an important marker for this disease.

> *Melanie was 17 when I first met her. She had a swollen knee which had been bothering her, off and on, for six years. This hadn't prevented her from trying to lead a normal life, and she was in fact a year ahead of her age group in school. What was remarkable was that she had done this despite being legally blind. Slowly and insidiously, beginning in her early teens, she had lost her vision.*

Up to a third of children with pauciarticular JIA are at high risk of 'silent' progressive eye damage, because of continuing low-grade inflammation in the front portion of the eye. The eye isn't red or painful, but the inflammation, called iridocyclitis, can cause cataracts, glaucoma, scarring of the cornea and loss of vision. The earliest signs can be detected only by careful examination by an eye specialist. Early detection, and the possibility of effective treatment, means that every child at risk must be followed carefully and frequently – at least annually into adulthood. The highest risk is within the first few years, and examinations should be more frequent then. Eye inflammation may occur, or progress, even if the joint disease is in remission.

Eye inflammation is most common with pauciarticular JIA, but it can occur (in up to 10 per cent) in children with other types of JIA. This means that all children with arthritis should be seen at least once by an eye specialist.

When older children develop pauciarticular arthritis, it may be an indication that they will go on to develop ankylosing spondylitis, the arthritis of inflammatory bowel disease or psoriatic arthritis. Unlike the younger children, who almost never have hip arthritis, hip inflammation is common in this group.

Arthritis involving many joints

About 20 per cent of children with arthritis have polyarticular disease. By definition, five or more joints are affected. The arthritis may look a great deal like adult rheumatoid arthritis (RA), and roughly half of these children will have a positive test for rheumatoid factor (RF). As in adult RA, a positive RF test tends to identify those who are not going to do well in the long term; those with RF-negative polyarthritis do much better.

Arthritis as part of Still's disease

A hundred years ago, George Frederic Still, a young English doctor in training, described the first cases of what has since become known as Still's disease. Children with this variant make up about a fifth of all cases of childhood arthritis.

These children are sick, and look sick. They have a systemic (i.e. involving many parts of the body) illness. High fevers, a blotchy red skin rash that comes and goes, enlarged lymph glands and a high white blood cell count often lead the doctor to search first for infection or childhood leukaemia. Arthritis tends to appear later, developing in about three-quarters of patients within 3 to 12 months.

Attacks with the systemic features are unpredictable, varying from a single episode to recurring episodes over a number of years. Usually, however, this aspect of Still's disease subsides within five years. The arthritis, however, continues as a progressive illness in about half the cases. The more joints are involved, and the earlier the age of onset of Still's, the poorer the long-term outlook for full functioning as an adult.

Children with Still's disease sometimes die, with liver disease and infection the most common causes of death. The heart may be involved, and heart failure can occur, particularly if there is severe anaemia as well. Most deaths occur within the first ten years of the illness.

What happens in the long run?

A significant minority of children – 30 to 50 per cent – experience abnormalities of growth. In many this seems to reflect the intense local inflammatory process. In the knee of a child of three or four, for example, the inflammation may provoke a 'growth spurt' of the adjacent bones, and that leg may be longer as a result. In an older child, the same stimulus may cause a brief growth spurt and then early bone fusion at the growth centre; because the opposite leg continues to grow, the affected leg will soon be shorter. Children who habitually don't use a leg because of pain may also develop growth retardation in that leg.

About a fifth of children will have 'micrognathia' (the jaw will be small and underdeveloped). Two patients I've been following since they were infants are now young women in their 20s; both have undergone jaw surgery to correct their 'receding chin' deformity and improve the way their teeth come together, and both are delighted with the result.

Children who are ill with Still's disease will experience slowing of their growth as long as the disease is active, so an experienced child rheumatologist will monitor growth very carefully. Growth retardation is also seen in children who are put on corticosteroids such as prednisone. Because these drugs can also cause osteoporosis in both children and adults, they are used only after careful consideration of the risks, and measures are taken to reduce those risks.

Remission of the arthritis

One of the cruel misconceptions about childhood arthritis is that the child will outgrow the disease. In fact, in just under half the children, the arthritis will continue past puberty.

The pattern of arthritis tends to stay the same over the years. Most of the children with pauciarticular arthritis will continue in that pattern; they have little disability and tend to do very well. For this group, vision is the big concern. However, some of them (about 15 per cent) will evolve into a polyarticular pattern and won't do so well. The change from pauciarticular to polyarticular arthritis, if it is going to occur, usually happens within the first five years.

Half the children who have polyarticular disease and are RF-negative will do well, and even go into permanent remission. Similarly, half of those with Still's disease will experience remission. The other half, along with those with RF-positive polyarticular disease, are not so lucky, and most will develop major difficulties with functioning as the years go by. A very small number of children with polyarticular disease will have their eyes affected, so they too should be closely watched. It is very rare for the eye to be affected in Still's disease.

How is childhood arthritis treated?

Exactly the same principles of treatment that we use in adult arthritis apply here. They include:

- suppression of inflammation,

- control of pain,

- maintenance of function,

- avoidance of complications.

Because the long-term outlook in an individual child can only be guessed at, treatment is long-term and involves many different types of therapists. Paediatric rheumatologists, physiotherapists, occupational therapists, social workers and the family doctor make up the core team. Eye specialists, orthopaedic surgeons, dietitians, psychologists and teachers are involved from time to time.

Methotrexate is the mainstay of treatment of JIA. Paediatric rheumatologists tend to use it in its injectable (subcutaneous) form, and have found it to be both effective and safe, even with prolonged use. Corticosteroid injections into the joint(s) are also very helpful, and in the child with pauciarticular arthritis may, with NSAIDs, be the only treatment needed. 'Biological' drugs, such as etanercept and infliximab, work well for many who do not respond to methotrexate, NSAIDs or 'combination' therapy as used in adult rheumatoid arthritis.

Dealing with childhood arthritis

Dr Helen Emery, a San Francisco paediatric rheumatologist, sets out the following important principles:

- Growth is a good indication of how well the disease is being controlled.

- It's easy to treat a chronically ill child like an infant, but it's wrong.

- Keep the child in school. Schooling at home is often second-rate, and socialisation suffers.

- Be aggressive with physiotherapy and occupational therapy. Be alert for joint contractures ('tightening up' at the joints, especially of knee and hip), and treat them early.

- Be aware of the effect of the illness on the child, the parents, brothers and sisters.

- Keep a balance. The child's life and the family's life should not revolve around the disease.

Finally, declares Dr Emery:

- A child goes in a wheelchair over my dead body.

Polymyositis and dermatomyositis

'Myositis' means inflammation of muscle. 'Dermato-' refers to an additional component of skin inflammation and 'poly-' means 'many'.

These two rare conditions – polymyositis is about twice as common as dermatomyositis – are similar, in terms of who's affected, to many of the other inflammatory diseases; women are more commonly affected and the age of onset is usually between 40 and 60. A small number of children also develop the condition.

Sometimes these conditions develop in people who have other 'connective tissue' diseases, particularly systemic lupus erythematosus. In a few patients, particularly those who are older when the symptoms develop, muscle inflammation may be a clue to an unsuspected cancer.

Signs and symptoms of polymyositis and dermatomyositis

The main symptom is muscle weakness. It usually comes on very slowly and is painless. At most, there is mild muscle aching. The muscles around the hips and the shoulders are those mainly affected. Patients have difficulty getting out of a chair or off the toilet. Climbing stairs becomes difficult. Holding the arms up to shampoo hair or to hang clothes on a line becomes impossible. The neck muscles may become weak, and swallowing may be difficult.

If a skin rash develops, we call the condition dermatomyositis. The rash can be extensive; it's reddish in colour, and in some areas there may be thickening and scaling of the skin – particularly on the backs of the hands, mainly over the knuckles. Around the eyes the skin may have a purplish colour.

Many patients will have systemic symptoms, such as fever, fatigue and weight loss. A number will have Raynaud's phenomenon – whitening of the fingers when exposed to cold. Shortness of breath may develop, due to one or more factors: the breathing muscles may be weak, there may be inflammatory scarring in the lungs and in some individuals the heart muscle itself is affected.

There has been a great deal of debate over whether the disease is linked to cancer. There is general consensus that it is, because cancer is more common in people with dermato/polymyositis than in people of similar background with rheumatoid arthritis, but not all researchers are convinced. In at least some instances polymyositis leads to discovery of a cancer, surgical removal results in marked improvement in the polymyositis and then the cancer and the polymyositis return together at a later date. The risk of cancer seems to be in the older age groups, especially in people with dermatomyositis. The cancer is usually obvious after a reasonable (not an exhaustive) investigation, and if it hasn't turned up within two to three years it probably won't.

Diagnosis

Diagnosis usually requires three separate approaches. Blood tests are done to detect raised levels of enzymes released from the inflamed muscles. Electromyography (insertion of a fine needle into the muscle to measure electrical activity) gives additional information. Finally, the most important test is a muscle biopsy. A small sample of muscle is removed, either by surgery or through a large needle, and examined under the microscope. The first two tests are needed because the inflammatory process may be 'patchy' (not evenly distributed in all muscles) and may come and go in intensity, so the muscle enzyme levels may sometimes be normal. The biopsy is done because there are other muscle diseases that may act the same but look different under the microscope and respond quite differently to treatment.

Treatment

Initially, patients are treated with corticosteroids, usually prednisone, in high doses. They often feel better soon after treatment is started, but it may take up to three months for full muscle strength to return. Patients should also be put on preventive treatment for osteoporosis. High-dose steroids must be continued for some time – at least until the muscle enzyme level drops to normal. Thereafter, the dose is slowly reduced. Not all patients respond to this treatment, however, and sometimes it's necessary to add either methotrexate or azathioprine. Recently, intravenous treatment with gamma-globulin has helped patients who still don't respond – but the only patient I used it on achieved little obvious benefit.

Outcome

Treatment has improved the outlook substantially over the last 40 years. People still die, though, from infection or as a result of lung or heart involvement. My personal experience has varied. I am currently following up two patients who have had the disease for well over 20 years. Both have stable but persisting weakness, and although they require continuing treatment they are able to live normal lives. I have had a number of patients whose treatment was stopped as they improved, and they remain well. But I have also had several patients whose polymyositis was linked to cancers that proved fatal.

Scleroderma (systemic sclerosis)

'Sclero-' means 'hard' and '-derma' refers to the skin. Scleroderma is a condition in which the skin is tight and thickened. Its other name – 'systemic sclerosis' – recognises the fact that this process doesn't just involve the skin. Other parts of the body can also be affected. The common denominator, in skin and elsewhere, seems to be excessive production of one of the body's 'building block' proteins, collagen.

This is a rare disease. Like many of the other so-called 'auto-immune' or 'connective tissue' disorders, it affects more women than men and tends to come on in their 30s and 40s.

Skin characteristics in scleroderma

Early on, the skin involved (generally the skin of the hands and feet, and often the skin of the face) may be reddened and puffy. This period is brief, however, and in typical scleroderma the skin soon becomes tight and shiny. The fingers and hands are particularly affected. Wrinkles, and even the fine hairs on the backs of fingers, disappear. The skin on the back of the fingers resists pinching. Tightness restricts finger movement, and it's difficult to straighten fingers fully or to make a fist. Fingertips are easily injured, and cracks may be slow to heal.

The extent of this change varies from person to person. In some it may be limited to the fingers and hand, in others it may involve the arm, face, trunk or legs. The process seems to spread from the fingers and toes, and move centrally.

Telangiectasia
Small blood vessels, normally invisible to the naked eye, often dilate enough to be apparent. Reddish 'freckles' that briefly turn pale when pressed are common, particularly on the face and palms.

Raynaud's phenomenon
Fingers (and sometimes toes) turn dead white and numb with exposure to cold, and then experience burning, flushing and tingling when rewarmed. Although Raynaud's is common in other conditions (and in up to 10 per cent of the general population),

here it is almost always present, probably reflecting the fact that circulation to the fingers is seriously reduced as part of the 'tightening' process.

Systemic involvement

Microscopic thickening and scarring of lung tissue
X-rays and pulmonary function tests show that well over half the patients with scleroderma do not have normal lungs. Many of them have no symptoms, but others experience shortness of breath, particularly with exercise.

The other lung complication that may develop is called 'pulmonary hypertension'. This isn't common but it is serious: the prolonged effort of pumping blood into the arteries of the lungs may overload the capacity of the heart, and heart failure can result.

Heartburn
Heartburn is one of the most common systemic symptoms of scleroderma. The muscle of the oesophagus (the passage from throat to stomach) becomes thin and weak, and is largely replaced by scar tissue. This means that swallowing is inefficient and occasionally difficult, and that the acid contents of the stomach frequently flow back up the oesophagus and cause pain.

Scleroderma can also affect other parts of the gut. Constipation or diarrhoea may become a problem.

Heart involvement
This is not often a symptom but there can be thickening of the membrane around the heart (the pericardium), and occasionally it's inflamed and causes pain (pericarditis). Actual heart muscle is rarely involved, although there may be patchy scarring. High blood pressure and pulmonary hypertension can tax the heart's ability to pump effectively.

Scleroderma of the kidney
This is also not very common but it is extremely serious. It often develops quite suddenly, with severe high blood pressure (hypertension) and kidney failure. The initial problem seems to occur in the small blood vessels of the kidney. They narrow, choking off

normal blood flow. This triggers a chemical release from the kidneys that causes severe hypertension. The high blood pressure in turn causes further kidney blood vessel damage, and the vicious circle continues.

What happens in the long term?

I diagnosed scleroderma in Jack four years ago and have been following him up ever since. Tightening and stiffening of his fingers and hands, along with Raynaud's phenomenon, were what first brought him to me. He was 56, the manager of a local farm co-op, and I was pleased that my initial examination turned up nothing that would suggest a serious complication. I was wary, however, realising that things could turn sour on fairly short notice. And that's exactly what happened.

Three days after I had checked him over, about a year into his illness, he was admitted to his local hospital with severe high blood pressure and kidney and heart failure. He was lucky: the problem was recognised immediately and he was transferred to the kidney unit and treated aggressively. He weathered the storm but not without a price. He is now on dialysis three times weekly. His quality of life is surprisingly good. He's working full time, and I suspect that in the not too distant future he'll be lined up for a kidney transplant.

Researchers at the University of Pittsburgh recently summarised their long (1972–1995) and intensive experience with scleroderma. Over two-thirds of their patients never developed severe organ involvement. The first three years seem to be critical. If severe organ damage did occur, survival at nine years dropped from 72 per cent to 38 per cent. But since 1972 there have been a number of treatment discoveries and the picture has changed. Drugs to deal with kidney crisis – the ACE inhibitors – have been introduced, and the nine-year survival following this complication has gone from 40 per cent to 68 per cent. Many patients never need dialysis, or need it only for a short while.

More recently a new oral treatment (bosentan) for pulmonary hypertension has been developed. It does not 'cure' the condition, but seems to slow significantly the process.

CREST

There is a form of localised scleroderma, known as CREST, which seems to have a better outlook. CREST is an acronym, and the letters stand for

Calcinosis – small calcium deposits, the size of clumps of salt crystals, scattered beneath the skin and detectable by X-ray

Raynaud's phenomenon

(O)**E**sophagus involvement

Sclerodactyly – hardening of the skin of the fingers (and often very little more; no skin hardening above the elbow is allowed under this definition)

Telangiectasia – the little red 'freckles' of dilated blood vessels

Individuals with CREST have a much lower risk of kidney involvement. Pulmonary hypertension, however, remains a definite concern.

Treatment of scleroderma

Studies at the University of Pittsburgh, USA, have strongly suggested that penicillamine, a drug that interferes with the maturation of collagen (the protein chains that bind the skin down), influences the disease favourably.

Researchers working with an experimental mouse model for scleroderma have succeeded in blocking excessive production of collagen by using an antibody to transforming-growth-factor-β1. TGF-β1 plays a role in the lung and the skin changes in scleroderma, and the researchers' findings may point the way to, for the first time, a truly effective treatment.

To date, however, no drug has been shown to unequivocally arrest the disease. There was some hope that methotrexate might be effective (it isn't) and we now know that corticosteroids may in fact accelerate kidney deterioration.

Lacking better means to identify early scleroderma – before it has had a chance to cause damage – and lacking the means to arrest it at that stage, we are left to deal with problems as they arise. This means:

- Paying attention to symptoms of shortness of breath and obtaining periodic tests of lung function.

- Watching carefully for the development of high blood pressure (which we can do something about).

- Using physiotherapy to attempt to prevent contractures (stiffening up of the joints, which prevents full movement).

- Dealing with heartburn with advice to avoid evening snacks and to raise the head of the bed on blocks; drugs such as omeprazole may be necessary.

- Minimising problems of reduced circulation to the hands and fingers by insisting on no smoking, encouraging warm mitts in the cold, and paying prompt attention to small nicks and cuts; occasionally, drugs such as calcium-channel blocking agents marginally improve the finger circulation and help relieve the most intense symptoms of Raynaud's phenomenon.

Sjögren's syndrome (sicca syndrome)

Dryness of the eyes and mouth may reflect ageing and the use of certain medications (particularly antidepressants). It is also a common feature of many of the autoimmune diseases, including rheumatoid arthritis, systemic lupus erythematosus and scleroderma, where the dryness reflects inflammatory scarring of the glands that make lubricating tears and saliva.

This dryness often makes for intolerable eye itching or 'grittiness'. I often get my first clue that Sjögren's (pronounced 'show-grins') is a problem when patients volunteer that they use lubricating eye drops every day. I then ask if they keep a glass of water on the bedside table, if they wake up with their tongue stuck to the roof of the mouth, and if they can chew and swallow a soda cracker without washing it down with a drink.

There are also situations where the inflammatory scarring of these glands seems to be unconnected to any other disease. In those cases, we speak of 'primary' Sjögren's syndrome.

Primary Sjögren's syndrome may have a variety of symptoms other than dryness. These include:

- Episodic or persistent swelling of the parotid glands (the main source of saliva). These are located just in front of the ears, and swelling gives the cheeks a 'chipmunk' look.

- Muscle and joint pains, and even joint swelling that may resemble rheumatoid arthritis but does not result in cartilage or bone damage.

- Raynaud's phenomenon.

It has been discovered that a small number of people with primary Sjögren's syndrome (not those whose dryness is linked to other forms of arthritis) develop a form of lymph gland cancer. This is quite uncommon but does mean that periodic follow-up visits are a good idea.

As in secondary Sjögren's syndrome – related to other arthritic conditions – the treatment of primary Sjögren's is symptomatic. 'Artificial tears', mouth lubricants, and sugar-free gum and lemon drops help relieve dryness. Pilocarpine – a drug that stimulates the remaining glandular tissue to produce tears and saliva – is sometimes surprisingly effective. Careful attention to dental hygiene is important. Joint pain and swelling, and Raynaud's phenomenon, are also dealt with in their own right.

6
What's Going On?
A Guide to Symptoms

Patients with arthritis are often concerned about a new problem. Sometimes they can see a connection to their arthritis but often they can't.

The following are some of the more common, or more important, symptoms that are linked to arthritis, organised by the areas where they tend to crop up. Some occur in many different kinds of arthritis, some are very disease-specific. Some are also found in people who are otherwise quite healthy.

Head and neck

- headache
- scalp tenderness
- skin rash
- dry eyes (and often mouth)
- red, sometimes painful, eyes
- changes in vision
- ear pain
- pain with chewing
- hoarseness and/or pain with swallowing
- neck pain

Headache

Headache is common as a symptom of neck arthritis, especially rheumatoid arthritis (RA) and osteoarthritis (OA). It's usually felt at the back of the skull, and may spread forward up and over the scalp to the sides and front. A good physiotherapist can help with advice, especially regarding neck support at night, the way to use ice and gentle movement exercises. Sometimes gentle traction and even local corticosteroid injection may be necessary.

Scalp tenderness

When headache is coupled with scalp tenderness, the tenderness may be a clue to localised inflammation of one of the scalp blood vessels. This is called temporal (or 'giant cell') arteritis; it's related to polymyalgia rheumatica and is potentially very serious. The headache is usually very localised, and is usually in the area of the temple. Tenderness when combing or brushing the hair may be the symptom that is most troublesome. In the most severe cases, inflammation of another artery, the one providing blood to the visual nerve, may cause sudden loss of vision.

Skin rash

This is common in two kinds of arthritis. A red and sometimes scaling rash over the bridge of the nose, frequently much worse after being out in the sun, is characteristic of systemic lupus erythematosus (SLE). An itching, scaling, reddish rash in the hair at the back of the scalp – often ignored for years as 'dandruff' – or behind the ears, or in the ear canal, may be the only proof that someone with a single swollen joint has psoriatic arthritis.

Dry eyes

Eye dryness leading to an itchy, 'gritty' feeling is characteristic of Sjögren's syndrome. This happens in roughly 25 per cent of people with RA but is also seen in other arthritic conditions, including SLE. It happens just as often in people who have no arthritis. Dryness occurs because the tear gland of the eye is affected by low-grade inflammation, and tear production drops.

Particular care has to be taken of the cornea, the clear membrane covering the pupil. It's much more easily scratched, especially by contact lenses, and if that happens it can become infected. 'Artificial tears', which can be bought at any chemist shop, help restore lubrication to the eye but they are never as good as the real thing.

People with Sjögren's syndrome (or 'sicca syndrome') often also notice marked dryness of the mouth and, in the case of women, the vagina. Many patients use sugarless lemon drops or gum to stimulate saliva. I've never been very impressed with artificial mouth lubricants, but in the last few years a drug that stimulates the remaining glands to produce their own lubricant – pilocarpine – has become available in tablet form. I've been quite pleased with its effectiveness. Finally, without the protection of normal saliva the teeth are very vulnerable to cavities. It's important to brush and floss daily, and to get regular dental check-ups. The teeth can be protected by special applications of a fluoride solution.

Red, sometimes painful, eyes

These may be a sign of significant corneal damage in Sjögren's syndrome. They may also occur in RA (where the eye is usually painless) or in the seronegative forms of spondylarthritis (such as ankylosing spondylitis and psoriatic arthritis), where they may be quite irritable. Photophobia (discomfort from bright lights) can be a real problem. Red eyes tend to clear up, though an eye specialist should probably be consulted, especially if pain or blurring of vision occurs.

Changes in vision

These are uncommon. Those that complicate the red eyes mentioned above tend to occur slowly. Even slower to develop is the 'silent' loss of vision seen in some forms of childhood (juvenile chronic) arthritis – which is why monitoring by an eye specialist is so important. A sudden loss of vision, or double vision or blurring of vision, is a serious symptom of temporal arteritis. Antimalarial drugs should never lead to vision changes if taken as prescribed, although the eyes should still be checked by an eye specialist at least twice a year. Much more likely is the possibility of 'speeded-up' development of cataracts when patients are on long-term corticosteroid treatment.

Ear pain

This pain usually isn't from the ear itself. It may arise from arthritis in the jaw joint (temporo-mandibular joint, or TMJ) but is much more commonly from inside the mouth (such as an abscessed tooth) or the throat.

Pain with chewing

If pain is felt just in front of the ear, it's almost certainly coming from the TMJ. If, however, a patient tells me that the pain is in the temple region at the side of the skull, I think of temporal arteritis.

Hoarseness and/or pain with swallowing

Inflammatory arthritis – usually RA – can affect any joint in the body. That includes the tiny joints that anchor the vocal cords in the throat. Inflammation here can cause hoarseness, or pain in the throat with swallowing. This isn't common but it may cause a lot of worry. Inhalable corticosteroid sprays, normally used in the treatment of asthma, are the most effective way to settle down the inflammation.

Neck pain

Neck pain is very common – almost as common as low back pain. It comes on suddenly, causes severe pain with movement, responds to an ice pack and neck support (with a firm collar or soft 'ruff') and clears up within days to a few weeks. Unlike low back pain, I would not recommend chiropractic manipulation for neck pain.

Most neck pain, though, spills over into the surrounding tissues, either up the back of the skull or down into the shoulder region. Neck pain may be referred from somewhere else, such as the heart. Heart attack pain, and similar referred pain, tends to be felt in the front or sides of the neck, whereas true neck pain tends to be felt in the muscles in the back of the neck.

A word about X-rays: just about everyone over the age of 40 will have a 'terrible-looking neck' on X-ray. Don't take such a diagnosis seriously. If there is significant neck disease, a careful examination, which is a far better test, will pick it up.

Chest

- chest pain
- heart pain
- breastbone pain
- cough and/or shortness of breath

Chest pain

Sharp, severe chest pain when breathing can be due to a 'muscle pull' or a fractured rib, but most commonly it's a sign of inflammation of the pleural membrane. This membrane (actually two) consists of a thin double layer of tissue that surrounds the lungs. A very small amount of fluid coats the inner layer, and allows it to move gently and smoothly within the outer layer as the lungs expand and shrink with each breath.

Inflammation between these layers is called 'pleurisy'. Usually pleurisy is a symptom of lung infection, but it can also occur in arthritis – particularly in RA and SLE. If it does happen and causes pain, treatment, usually with a brief course of cortico-steroids, will settle things down.

Heart pain

'Crushing' chest pain, felt front and centre and sometimes also in the neck, jaw and/or left arm, is well known as the typical pain of a heart attack. What isn't so well known is that pericarditis (inflammation of the double-layered membrane that encloses the heart) can provoke pain that is identical.

The typical story goes something like this: 'Right now I'm not having pain unless I cough or take a very deep breath, but last night I was really frightened. I woke up and it felt like someone was standing right in the middle of my chest. My jaw ached, and

my left arm felt heavy and had a dull ache, too. I felt really short
of breath and sat up. That seemed to help the pain, but each time
I lay back it got worse again.'

Like pleurisy, pericarditis can be part of the inflammation of
arthritis, and it usually happens in someone with either RA or
SLE. Again, corticosteroids, and sometimes NSAIDs, are helpful
in relieving inflammation and pain.

Pericarditis does not mean that the heart has been damaged.

Breastbone pain

Inflammatory arthritis, especially RA, may cause pain in the
joints that connect the inner ends of the collar-bones (the clavi-
cles) to the breastbone (the sternum). Pain and swelling will
be noted on either side of the windpipe (the trachea) just as
it disappears below the sternum. There is also a joint (the
manubrio-sternal joint) in the breastbone, about three finger-
breadths below the notch where the windpipe disappears, which
can become inflamed. Finally, on either side of the sternum,
where the ribs attach, tenderness (but not inflammation) is also
common, particularly in fibromyalgia.

Cough and/or shortness of breath

Many forms of inflammatory arthritis – particularly RA – and
many of the less common connective tissue disorders (such as
dermatomyositis and scleroderma) can affect the lungs.
Microscopic scarring can occur, leading to shortness of breath
with exertion and, often, a dry cough. Sometimes the problem is
due to a build-up of fluid in the space between the two layers of
tissue that surround the lung.

Shortness of breath is not a common symptom in arthritis, and
it is always necessary to investigate it fully to be sure it isn't due
to some other cause, such as infection. Some of the drugs used to
treat arthritis may also turn out to be the culprit, so this symptom, although quite unusual in arthritis, should be reported to the
doctor.

Abdomen

- difficulty swallowing
- heartburn
- cramps, diarrhoea
- black or bloody bowel movements

Difficulty swallowing

Swallowing problems aren't common – if you don't count trying to get down all the pills some of you have to take each day. For that, it's useful to remember to swallow standing up, and to wash the pills down with a second glass of water.

If the muscles that control swallowing are carefully studied, using special techniques, muscle weakness or incoordination can be discovered in quite a number of people with some of the connective tissue disorders, particularly scleroderma (SLE and inflammatory muscle diseases are also in this category). This can lead to a feeling that food is 'catching' behind the breastbone.

Heartburn

Heartburn (or 'reflux oesophagitis') is the symptom of burning felt behind the breastbone, sometimes associated with a sour acid taste. It is particularly a problem at night, especially if the person has eaten late in the evening. Sometimes the person awakens choking. The acid stomach contents have not only come back up the oesophagus (the 'swallowing tube') from the stomach but have also spilled into the upper part of the breathing passages. Spasm of the larynx is brief but can be very frightening.

This can be a problem for many people without arthritis, particularly those who are overweight or pregnant. But the same muscle incoordination of the oesophagus that slows swallowing in some forms of arthritis may also affect the valve at the opening of the oesophagus into the stomach. This too allows 'acid reflux' to occur.

The most effective treatment is to avoid food in the evening. Raising the head of the bed on 15cm (6-inch) blocks, or placing a foam wedge under the mattress to raise the upper body, will work, but both are awkward. Sometimes a prescription medication to reduce stomach acid and improve the action of the valve is called for. Ranitidine seems to work well for most people.

Cramps, diarrhoea

These aren't usually symptoms of arthritis, unless there is an underlying problem of ulcerative colitis or Crohn's disease. Much more likely is the possibility that the problems are caused by medication. These symptoms should be reported to your doctor. If this isn't immediately possible, the next dose of the arthritis medicine (except corticosteroids) should be skipped until there has been an opportunity to sort out the problem.

Black or bloody bowel movements

A bit of blood on the toilet paper is common and is usually a sign of unimportant bleeding, such as from a 'pile', or haemorrhoid. But black bowel movements – assuming you haven't been taking iron pills or stomach medicines (e.g. Pepto-Bismol) that contain bismuth, which create this effect – mean significant bleeding from higher up in the gastrointestinal tract. The most common source is an ulcer in either the stomach or the small intestine. The usual cause for this, in patients with arthritis, is medication – usually an NSAID.

Recognisable blood, either bright or dark red, usually means that the bleeding is from lower down, often in the large intestine. However, if a stomach ulcer is bleeding briskly, the blood may travel down the intestinal tract so quickly that it doesn't have time to be chemically changed to the black colour.

Whatever the cause, black or bloody bowel movements mean trouble. Get medical attention quickly.

Genitals

- discharge from the penis
- blood in the urine
- vaginal symptoms

Discharge from the penis

There are two situations where discharge from the penis can be linked to arthritis. Gonorrhoea, one of the sexually transmitted diseases, can cause an acute arthritis. The appearance of a hot and swollen joint (often a wrist or knee) may in fact be the first indication that the symptoms of burning on urination and the slight discharge from the penis were important.

Reactive arthritis is discussed more fully in Chapter 2. It, too, can be triggered by a sexually transmitted disease, such as infection with *Chlamydia*, and a discharge from the penis can precede its development.

Blood in the urine

When blood is detected in the urine, it's usually microscopic blood, found in the course of a routine urine test; the urine sample is clear to the naked eye. When the urine is visibly pink or red, the bleeding is usually from the bladder, prostate, urethra or vagina, and is not related to either arthritis or its treatment. The one exception is an unusual one – when gout is complicated by the formation of kidney stones. Then the bleeding is invariably accompanied by 'terrible' knife-like pain in the flank. This pain often spreads round from the back to the lower abdomen and into the groin. In men, it's often felt into the testicle.

Vaginal symptoms

Vaginal symptoms are not often related to arthritis. Vaginal dryness, which is common as part of Sjögren's syndrome, and vaginal ulcerations, which occasionally appear in SLE, are two exceptions. Gonorrhoea, in women as in men, may cause an acute inflammatory arthritis, but it doesn't usually cause distinctive vaginal symptoms.

Lymph nodes

Swollen 'glands' in the neck, armpits and groin are often discovered accidentally. They don't usually cause discomfort. There are, of course, many reasons why lymph nodes become enlarged, and their discovery should be pointed out to your doctor. They are surprisingly common in RA, and are almost always benign. Nevertheless, enlarged lymph nodes may be an important sign of a completely different problem and should not be ignored.

Shoulder, arm and hand

- shoulder and arm pain
- elbow pain, lumps and swellings
- wrist pain at the base of the thumb
- numbness in the hands
- fingers that 'lock'
- the suddenly droopy finger
- white fingers
- 'funny' fingernails

Shoulder and arm pain

There are several possible causes of shoulder pain but it usually isn't too hard to work out the cause of most. It is important to get a precise description of the location of the pain itself, and then some idea of what makes it better or worse.

A principle that's important to remember: if the pain isn't affected by movement of the shoulder, it's probably coming from somewhere else.

Pain originating in the bones, muscles or nerves of the neck
This pain is felt in the muscles on top of the shoulder, between the base of the neck and the end of the collarbone. It can also radiate upward into the back of the skull. If shoulder pain of this type is felt on one side only, it is almost certainly 'mechanical' and not inflammatory in origin. If it involves both sides, either category is possible. If there's pressure on one of the nerves as it exits between the bones of the neck, shoulder pain will track down the arm, and it can be accompanied by tingling or weakness in the arm and hand. Pain of this type will be aggravated by movement

of the head and neck, and sometimes made better by such unusual 'tricks' as placing the hand on top of the head.

Pain originating at the outside end of the collarbone

Pain in the acromio-clavicular joint – that is, where the outer end of the collarbone links up with the shoulder blade – is quite localised to that joint. You can feel the joint by tracing the collarbone out toward the point of the shoulder; it's just before the 'bump' of the acromion (the bone that forms the tip of the shoulder), and you can identify it by rotating your arm at the shoulder joint. If this joint is the problem, the pressure of your finger will cause pain, and you may feel a 'grinding' as the shoulder moves around.

Pain from the shoulder joint itself, or from the 'rotator cuff'

Pain is often felt not in the shoulder but in the upper outer arm, about 7.5cm (3 inches) below the tip of the shoulder. The pain here is much worse if the arm is raised sideways to the horizontal, and may be so sharp that lowering the arm slowly back down is impossible. Halfway down, if there is a tear or a painful focus in the tendons and ligaments that surround it (the 'rotator cuff'), you will be forced to let the arm fall limply to your side. Shoulder pain of this type can usually be traced to inflammation of a bursa (see below) or tendon just beneath the acromion. It is common in many forms of arthritis but is even more common in 'normal' people. There isn't much room between the acromion and the head of the humerus (the part of the arm bone that links up to form the shoulder joint), and shoulder movement narrows the gap even more. Shoulder tendons, and the bursa that cushions them, fill this gap and are easily inflamed by overuse. Pain is particularly bad at night. NSAIDs, and in resistant cases local corticosteroid injections, usually settle the problem.

Pain 'referred' to the arm or shoulder from somewhere else

Referred pain is characteristically from a source deep in the body. The brain has difficulty 'reading' its source, and is tricked by the nervous system into mislabelling it. The best-known example is the pain when the supply of oxygen to the heart is insufficient. The pain of angina is often felt as a deep ache in the entire left arm, worse with excitement or exertion and better with rest. Pain from the part of the abdomen beneath the diaphragm may be felt on top of the shoulder, just above the shoulder blade. This may, in fact, be the first sign of a gall bladder attack.

Elbow pain, lumps and swellings

The two outer bumps at the elbow are the epicondyles. The bump in the middle (at the point of the elbow) is the olecranon. Elbow pain may be due to joint disease but the most common cause is *epicondylitis*. When it's on the outside of the elbow the popular term is 'tennis elbow', and when it's on the inside the term is 'golfer's elbow'. Pain is felt at, or just below, one of the bony bumps at the elbow; if the elbow is tender, bursitis (see below) may be the problem.

There's some argument as to what is actually going on but there's no disagreement as to the location. Pain arises in the area where the forearm muscle tendons attach to the elbow. In the case of 'tennis elbow' the muscles are those that brace the wrist when you make a tight fist or grip something tight (as in holding a tennis racket). The opposing muscles, those that hold the wrist in the slightly bent position, cause pain on the inside of the elbow when contracted. Age (over 40) and overuse (most cases are not caused by tennis or golf) are felt to be the main factors in development of epicondylitis. There have been over 40 different treatments proposed, but the injection of corticosteroid clears up the symptoms in almost everyone. To be honest, however, most patients (if willing to be patient) will recover on their own within the next 12 months.

In addition to swelling of the elbow joint itself (which makes it impossible to fully bend or straighten the arm), there are at least two fairly common types of swelling in this region (Figure 6.1):

- bursitis (inflammation of a bursa),
- rheumatoid nodules.

A bursa is a small, collapsed sac containing a few drops of lubricating fluid – think of an uninflated balloon. The body has many bursae, which lie particularly at pressure points where they cushion the skin from being damaged by local injury. The olecranon bursa sits under the skin just below the tip of the elbow, at

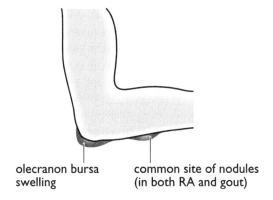

olecranon bursa
swelling

common site of nodules
(in both RA and gout)

Figure 6.1 Common swellings of the elbow region

the point where we usually rest our elbows on the arms of a chair. The accumulation of fluid can swell the 'balloon', and then the bursa can be felt as quite puffy and sometimes tense.

Sudden swelling is painful. It can be caused by injury (a fall on an icy pavement), inflammation (gout can do it) or infection. If there is any doubt, check it out with your doctor.

Slower swelling is usually painless. The bursa is less puffy but it's constantly getting in the way. This type of swelling has a number of possible causes. Local injury is probably the most common. It's very often seen, however, in RA.

It's usual to make sure that infection isn't the problem. If there's any doubt, a sample of fluid is drained off through a needle and sent to the lab. Once infection has been ruled out, the bursa is left alone. If local injury caused it, it will go down on its own. Cortisone injections tend to speed up the process and have been used where RA is the cause, with some success and some failures. If the bursa doesn't settle down then, and its size is a problem, it is sometimes removed surgically.

Rheumatoid nodules are similar in that they can be removed but will often return. They are most often found just below the elbow, on the forearm where it rests on the arms of a chair. Such nodules can develop in a number of other locations – all it takes is RA (and usually rheumatoid factor) and pressure. Nodules on fingers, over knuckles or where a pencil or a hammer is held tightly, and on the back of the heel where the shoe or boot rubs, are almost as common. They are usually small – pea-sized or less.

Wrist pain at the base of the thumb

There are two sources of pain here. One is OA between one of the wrist bones and the thumb metacarpal. This is common, particularly in the non-dominant hand (in most of us, the left hand). It shows up as aching, and sharp pain with tight gripping, and in time a bony lump often develops over this joint. Local cortisone injection, a thumb splint or, very rarely, surgery are ways to deal with this.

The other source of pain is de Quervain's tenosynovitis – inflammation of the tendon that pulls the thumb back in a 'hitch-hiking' position. NSAIDs and splinting may help, but if the inflammation persists a local cortisone injection may be needed.

Numbness in the hands

About 1 in every 1,000 adults has this problem at any given time. The usual story is something like this:

> *'What's wrong with my hand? I'm waking up every night with burning pain in my fingers. They feel numb, especially my thumb and the next three fingers. If I hang my arm over the side of the bed, or shake my hand hard, the numbness improves and I can get back to sleep. It comes on during the day, too, especially if I'm holding up a newspaper or gripping the steering wheel for a long time.'*

The diagnosis here is 'carpal tunnel syndrome', and the problem is pressure on the median nerve at the wrist (see Figure 6.2). The median nerve is responsible for sensation in the palm side of the thumb and the first three fingers. This nerve also causes the muscle in the palm, at the base of the thumb, to contract.

Pressure can be due to many things, including some that have nothing to do with arthritis (pregnancy and low thyroid function are just two). But in my practice, RA is the most common cause. Pressure on the median nerve is caused by inflammatory swelling of the tissues at the wrist that lie just beneath the nerve. The nerve gets trapped between this swollen tissue and the tough ligament that crosses above it. When the nerve is injured in this fashion, it hurts.

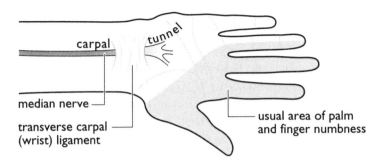

Figure 6.2 Wrist anatomy in carpal tunnel syndrome

An occupational therapist can provide the patient with a carpal tunnel splint to wear at night. This keeps the wrist from bending and putting even more pressure on the nerve.

If symptoms are really severe and medical management seems to be ineffective, surgery is recommended. (If symptoms persist for too long, the nerve can be permanently damaged.) Pressure can be relieved permanently by a relatively simple surgical procedure, 'carpal tunnel release', which involves cutting the restraining ligament. This can often be done on an out-patient basis, the patient going home the same day.

Fingers that 'lock'

Rheumatologists call this a 'trigger finger'. It's fairly common, and is due to inflammatory thickening on one of the tendons that bend the fingers. This thickening, like a knot in a rope, blocks the smooth flow of the tendon as the finger muscles contract. The knot gets stuck, or catches on corners. This is easy to treat. An injection of a corticosteroid in the thickened area usually frees things up.

The suddenly droopy finger

The extensor tendons of the fingers (those on the back of the hand, which allow us to point fingers at others) pass through some tissue at the back of the wrist called the 'tenosynovial sheath'. This tissue is often inflamed, swollen and painful in RA, and the inflammation can thin and weaken the tendons. A sudden 'ping', a sharp pain, and a finger droops. Considering how common this type of swelling is, it's surprising that tendon rupture doesn't happen more often. Sometimes a surgeon removes the inflamed tissue if wrist pain on finger movement suggests that tendon rupture is likely. Usually, however, surgery occurs after the event. The tendon is reattached or replaced and the inflammatory tissue removed.

White fingers

The story here is usually 'Every time I go out in the cold without my gloves, my fingers go white. I lose the feeling in them. When I warm them up they go purple, then fiery red, and they burn for several minutes'. Sometimes the simple act of scrubbing potatoes under the cold-water tap, or jumping into the North Sea in July, will have the same effect.

This is Raynaud's phenomenon. It's very common, particularly in young women. Approximately 10 per cent of the population report Raynaud's symptoms, and most of the time they don't signify an underlying problem. Raynaud's can, however, be part of SLE, or some other connective tissue diseases such as scleroderma. The phenomenon is usually little more than an annoyance, but if it's a problem drugs called 'calcium channel blocking agents' can help make it more tolerable.

'Funny' fingernails

The nail changes of psoriasis have been mentioned in Chapter 2.

The nail fold (the ridge of skin along the sides and base of the fingernail) can have 'nail-fold vasculitis' in RA and sometimes in SLE. At first glance this can look like a hangnail – a tiny brown–black splinter at the edge of the nail. But these are not hangnails, and they tend to occur in crops, several fingers showing the same thing at the same time. They are probably similar in origin to the rheumatoid nodule, the result of a combination of rheumatoid inflammation in a tiny blood vessel and local pressure. They are harmless, and tend to come and go.

Hip, leg and foot

- hip and leg pain
- kneecap aching (patello-femoral syndrome)
- knee lumps and swellings
- calf pain and/or swelling
- heel pain
- foot numbness
- pain in the ball of the foot

Hip and leg pain

Pain from the lower back and sacroiliac joints
This is often 'referred' to the buttock and the back of the upper thigh. It's not sciatic pain, and doesn't mean that there is nerve pressure. This type of referred pain is often described as 'dull' or 'stiff', and lacks the severity of true sciatica. This location is typical for both ordinary mechanical low back pain and the pain of inflammation, as in ankylosing spondylitis.

If the pain continues below the back of the knee into the calf, sciatica is a distinct possibility. Pain here is caused by pressure on the root of one of the nerves as it leaves the spinal canal to pass down the leg. Sciatic pain is usually not 'deep and dull', but sharp and severe. It's often worse with coughing or straining to have a bowel movement and is usually, but not always, made better by lying down.

Pain similar in location – down the back of the thigh and calf – but less intense, and coming on with prolonged standing or walking, is characteristic of 'spinal stenosis' (see the section 'Low back pain' in Chapter 4).

Pain from problems in blood supply
Another significant leg pain is the pain of peripheral vascular disease or 'hardening of the arteries'. If the main blood vessels into the legs become narrowed by cholesterol deposits, pain may be the first symptom. It's usually felt in the calf. The person experiences a severe cramp that causes him or her to sit and rest, and

after a minute or two the walk can be resumed. (This kind of pain is called 'claudication', after the Roman emperor Claudius, although his leg pain wasn't due to bad circulation.)

Pain from irritation of the trochanteric bursa

On the side of the hip, right where we experience the maximum pressure when we lie on our side in bed, is a bony bump called the 'greater trochanter'. Because this is a pressure point, like the elbow, there is a bursa over this bump, and it can become very tender. Attaching to the upper surface of this bump is the tendon of the buttock muscle that helps keep the pelvis level when we walk – the tendon of the gluteus medius muscle – and this tendon can also become inflamed and painful. Finally, there is a tough sheet of tissue covering the outside of the thigh muscle, from pelvis to knee, known as the 'lateral (or 'iliotibial') band'. In middle age it can become very tight and tender, particularly where it passes over the trochanter.

Tenderness in these structures – trochanteric bursa, gluteus medius tendon and iliotibial band – is common and almost invariably provokes worry that there is something wrong with the hip – which is usually not the case.

Reassurance, stretching exercises and often a local injection of a mixture of corticosteroid and anaesthetic usually settle things down.

Pain from the hip joint

This is usually felt in the groin, spreading down the front of the thigh toward the knee. Some patients have pain only in the knee area, and it isn't until the doctor tries to move their hips that the true source is discovered. True hip pain is very rarely felt on the side of the hip or deep in the buttock.

Thigh numbness

Burning numbness of the upper thigh, overlapping the front and side, is due to pressure on a small nerve – the lateral femoral cutaneous nerve – usually just where it enters the leg at the outer groin. It is seen in association with pregnancy, obesity and hernia repair surgery.

Kneecap aching (patello-femoral syndrome)

Kneecap pain is typically described as 'deep and aching' and is felt over the front (or front and inner) aspect of the kneecap. It's made worse by going up or down stairs. Sitting in one position for some time is difficult. Women seem to have this symptom more than men, either in their teens or in later middle age. Very often the patient can feel a fine 'grating' by cupping the kneecap with the palm of the hand while bending and straightening the knee.

Hamstring muscle stretching, strengthening of the quadriceps muscle at the front of the thigh and sometimes taping the kneecap are the usual treatments. Time, and avoidance of things that make the pain worse, helps too.

Knee lumps and swellings

There are a number of bursae around the knee, but the one that most commonly 'blows up' is the pre-patellar bursa. This condition is called 'housemaid's knee', because of the traditional cause – kneeling. However, those I've seen in the past few years have been due to infection more than to local trauma.

Occasionally other bursae in the knee region will swell. Swelling just below the kneecap is called 'jumper's knee', and a very common one at the back of the knee is discussed below.

The other cause of swelling just below the kneecap is inflammation of the site where the tendon from the kneecap attaches to the shin. This site of attachment is called the tibial tubercle, and it can be felt as a bony bump. Inflammation here, like 'jumper's knee', is most often a problem in young male athletes. It's called Osgood–Schlatter's disease, and it gets better.

Calf pain and/or swelling

This symptom, which may come on very suddenly and look just like phlebitis in the calf, is actually due to arthritis in the knee. Behind the knee is a small fluid-filled sac called a 'popliteal bursa' or 'Baker's cyst' (see Figure 6.3). Normally it's very small and inapparent, but if the knee becomes inflamed and swells, the fluid from the swelling can leak backward and swell up the sac. If this happens slowly, over several days to weeks (which is

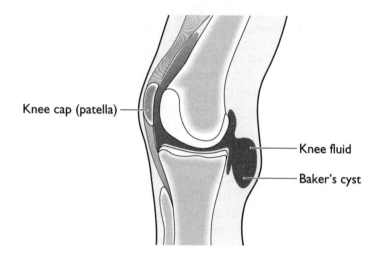

Knee cap (patella)

Knee fluid

Baker's cyst

Figure 6.3 Baker's cyst. Build-up of fluid in the knee can cause a Baker's cyst, a swelling behind the knee

the usual case), the main symptom is usually a sensation of fullness behind the knee, as if a ping-pong ball has been placed there.

But if the cyst fills up rapidly, its wall can be stretched thin and it can get very large like a balloon. With nowhere to go, it works its way down into the calf, where it can cause quite a bit of pain, particularly if the balloon breaks.

Treatment is directed toward the cause by injecting the knee with cortisone, which takes down the knee inflammation, and the cyst deflates.

Heel pain

A few years ago, on the first day of a hiking holiday, I awoke and attempted to stand. The moment my left heel made contact with the floor I felt an excruciating pain. I went hiking anyway, but my heel didn't touch the ground at any time. It was a dumb thing to do. The next day my heel was better but my calf was unbearable.

That was my one brief brush with plantar fasciitis. Pain here is usually caused by some form of overuse. The other setting in which it's common is the seronegative forms of spondylarthritis, such as ankylosing spondylitis. Treatment may be a problem, with pain persisting despite NSAIDs and proper insole padding. On occasion I have resorted to local cortisone injections. A special splint can be made, designed to stretch the tight tissues on the sole of the foot while the patient sleeps, but it's expensive.

The other site of pain is at the back of the heel, where the Achilles tendon attaches. Irritation here can be caused by overuse, tight tissues or inflammation. This is one tendon that I would never inject with corticosteroid. It carries enormous loads, and if the injection were to weaken the tendon it would be more likely to rupture than any other tendon in the body.

Foot numbness

Not too commonly, the small nerves of the foot will become 'trapped' at the ankle or between the bones at the ball of the foot. If symptoms of numbness or burning are severe, surgical release of the tissues pressing on the nerves is possible.

There are two other causes of foot numbness. Nerve pressure from higher up, often linked to sciatica, is one. The other is a 'sensory neuropathy', in which the smaller nerves that carry feelings of pressure and pain (from the skin to the spinal cord) are damaged. This can be caused by diabetes and RA but, because there are so many different possibilities, a full investigation is usually wise. Typically, the numbness is felt in the foot and ankle in a 'stocking' distribution.

Pain in the ball of the foot

Pain under the ball of the foot, where the toes attach, is called metatarsalgia. The 'ball', the thickened ridge running the width of the forefoot, is formed by the MTP joints (the joints that allow us to wiggle our toes) with a thick layer of padding (mostly fatty tissue) between the joint and the skin.

Metatarsalgia is common, sometimes as a result of the thinning of the fat pad that often comes with age, but more often as a result of inflammatory arthritis, particularly RA (see Figure 6.4). Inflammation here is painful, and damages the joints. This is often linked to the big toe twisting over, causing the second toe to ride up. The deformity at the base of the big toe is called a bunion.

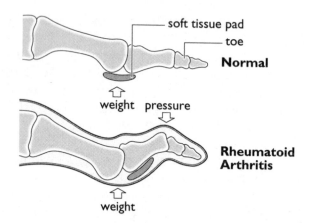

Figure 6.4 Common changes in the foot in rheumatoid arthritis. In RA the weight-bearing soft tissue cushion of the foot commonly migrates forward and the toe slips upward.

The result, often, is toes that overlap or toes that ride up – so-called 'cock-up' or 'hammer' toes. These deformities are due to a combination of inflammation, body weight and constricting footwear. Treatment should include suppressing inflammation, but, because a 100 per cent result is not always possible, the role of footwear should be considered.

'Walking shoes', built along the lines of the modern running shoe, are great. They have a neutral heel, sharing weight evenly between front and back, and provide excellent ankle and instep support. They are well padded, and all have lots of room for the occupational therapist to make an insole to shift the weight off the MTPs.

Back

- sudden back pain
- night pain

Sudden back pain

Sudden back pain is never good news. Usually it's simply an attack of 'acute mechanical low back pain' and will be better in a few days to weeks, but it can be quite incapacitating until this happens.

If the pain is higher than the 'low back' (what people refer to as 'the small of the back'), particularly up between the shoulder blades, a compression fracture of a vertebra (or vertebrae) is a possibility. There are several causes of compression fractures including infection and malignancy, but osteoporosis is high on the list.

Pain coming from deep in the belly – from the stomach, kidney or pancreas, or even from the main blood vessel, the aorta – can be felt in the back. Because there are so many possible sources, some of them serious, sudden back pain requires a full assessment by a competent doctor without delay.

Night pain

Night pain is also, in general, never good news. Ordinary back pain gets better with rest. Night back pain may be due to inflammation, as in ankylosing spondylitis, but it's also a symptom of bone infection and bone tumours, both benign and malignant. Night pain, too, requires a very careful look by a doctor.

Skin

Bruises and 'lovebites'

Bruising of the skin is not a common problem in arthritis except where an older patient has been taking prednisone for some time. Here, bruises appear suddenly, particularly on the arms, without any known injury. The skin is often paper-thin, and easily torn. Prednisone, even in relatively small doses, causes thinning of the cushion of fat under the skin of the arms. The skin naturally thins with ageing, and corticosteroids increase this tendency. These changes all combine to predispose to skin tearing and bruising.

Bruises can also be a problem if the platelets, those blood cells very important in clotting, are reduced in numbers. This can arise as a result of disease, such as SLE, or as a side effect of treatment. Quite a number of drugs can do this.

Clusters of pinpoint bleeding (a 'lovebite' or 'hickey') can result from either disease or drugs. These are most frequent on the shins and should be brought to your doctor's attention.

Joint with unbearable pain

Infections love joints that have already been damaged. This is true in OA, in all types of chronic arthritis and in RA. Joint infection is rare, but it's serious.

Infection usually settles in a single joint, at least at first. The pain from the infection is different from and much worse than the usual pain of rheumatoid or osteoarthritis. It keeps you awake at night, and brings tears when the joint is moved. Fever or chills may be clues to the true nature of the problem, but may not appear at first. Pain like this demands that a needle be inserted into the joint and a specimen of fluid sent to the lab to determine whether an infection is present. Early treatment is essential. Not only can the joint be badly damaged; a delay in diagnosis may result in death.

7
The Treatment of Arthritis

Aspirin and its cousins – the NSAIDs

For a long time, aspirin (acetylsalicylic acid) was the only NSAID we had. The first modern NSAIDs were developed in the 1950s and 1960s, and since the 1980s the number available has grown incredibly; we can now chose from ibuprofen, salsalate, diclofenac, naproxen, ketoprofen, piroxicam, indometacin, sulindac and others. In the recent past, a new generation of NSAIDs – the COX-2 specific drugs – has been developed. These drugs differ from each other in a number of ways – chemically, how often they need to be taken each day, cost, side effects – but they are very similar in one way: *they all seem to be equally effective as anti-inflammatories*. None of the newer NSAIDs has been found to be superior to any other, or to aspirin itself, in treating the two most common problems: osteoarthritis and rheumatoid arthritis.

NSAIDs are the most commonly prescribed of all drugs in arthritis. Global sales, to an estimated 30 million people, exceed £1.25 billion each year. Most of these prescriptions are probably inappropriate. Patients and their doctors have been oversold on their supposed benefits. This is particularly true in older people. A recent review in the *British Medical Journal* says that 'about 24 million prescriptions a year are written for NSAIDs in the UK. Half of these are given to patients over the age of 60. At any one time about 15 per cent of elderly people are taking an NSAID.'

However, when prescribed appropriately, NSAIDs are useful because they have a dual action: they are anti-inflammatory, helping to suppress joint swelling, warmth and pain; and they are analgesic, with pain-killing properties separate from their anti-inflammatory action.

The following can be said about NSAIDs:

- their effectiveness varies with the kind of arthritis being treated;

- they are rarely enough by themselves;

- serious complications are uncommon, but can arise without warning;

- different people, even with the same problem, respond differently to the same NSAID.

How to swallow a pill

Patients with some types of arthritis, as well as older people, may have problems getting a pill from mouth to stomach. The muscle of the swallowing tube, the oesophagus, is often weak or uncoordinated. This means that the medication may, though the swallower doesn't know it, get stuck on the way down. This can happen to people with normal swallowing, too, especially with big pills. A pill that gets stuck may be very irritating to the lining of the oesophagus. Prolonged contact there can cause ulceration, bleeding and, in the long term, scarring.

To reduce the risk of pill injury to the oesophagus:

- if possible, get smaller pills, as big ones are more likely to get stuck;

- swallow when standing (or sitting) upright, and don't lie down right after taking the pill;

- take plenty of water – at least half a glass;

- if the pill is big, check with your pharmacist to see if it can be ground up and mixed with a semi-liquid such as apple sauce.

COX-1 and COX-2: what's the difference?

There was long thought to be just one kind of cyclo-oxygenase (COX). COX is an enzyme found in many body tissues; it is important in the manufacture of prostaglandins. Prostaglandins are known to be one of the major players in inflammation, and NSAIDs are thought to work because they block COX and, hence, the synthesis of prostaglandins. Unfortunately, prostaglandins also have very important roles – such as protecting the stomach against acid damage and ensuring that kidney blood flow is maintained. Until recently we've had to take the bad with the good; effective NSAID blocking of inflammation often brought with it stomach ulcers and kidney impairment.

We now know that there are two kinds of COX: COX-1 promotes stomach protection and kidney blood flow, and COX-2 promotes inflammation. All of the traditional NSAIDs block both COX-1 and COX-2 (though some block one more than the other). Recently a number of new NSAIDs, said to be 'specific' for COX-2 (and therefore theoretically free of ulcer side effects) have been developed – celecoxib and rofecoxib are two of these. Because they promised to eliminate the risk of stomach bleeding in people most at risk – the elderly – they were immediately popular, and captured a huge segment of the NSAID market. But concerns and questions remain:

- Like the older NSAIDs, there is still a problem with fluid retention, worsening kidney function, heart failure and hypertension in vulnerable patients (particularly those with problems in those areas already).

- The risk of serious stomach bleeding has not been eliminated. At best, it has been reduced.

- People who take low-dose aspirin for their heart as well as either kind of NSAID are at increased risk of a stomach bleed – and may also lose the heart- and stroke-protecting benefits of the aspirin.

- There is even a possibility that the newer COX-2-blocking drugs increase the risk of a heart attack, particularly in someone with a history of heart disease.

Choosing an NSAID

For the individual patient one NSAID often seems to be best. To find that one, a sequence of NSAIDs is prescribed for relatively brief trial periods of about 7 to 10 days each. By the time three or possibly four have been tried, the doctor has a pretty good idea of how much that patient is going to be helped by an NSAID, and which one is best. Trying more would waste time and money.

Ideally, the NSAID chosen will be cheap, well tolerated, easy to remember to take and effective. Few drugs meet all these criteria.

You can bleed from the stomach on any of the traditional NSAIDs, particularly if:

- you are older (the risk increases with age),

- you have had an ulcer before,

- you are taking high doses of one NSAID, or combining two,

- you are also taking a corticosteroid such as prednisone,

- you are on a blood-thinning drug (anticoagulant),

- you have a serious medical condition,

and, although this is less certain, if:

- you smoke cigarettes,

- you drink alcohol.

If one of my patients falls into one of the 'high risk' categories – particularly if they are over 65, have had a previous ulcer, are taking low-dose aspirin for their heart or a blood-thinning drug (such as warfarin) or prednisone – my first question is whether they should be taking an NSAID at all. Would paracetamol be just as effective for pain control? Would a slight increase in prednisone be just as effective? Would a cortisone injection settle the problem? Only if the answer is 'no' would I, somewhat reluctantly, consider an NSAID. I would probably combine it with medication to reduce stomach acid (such as omeprazole) or increase stomach lining resistance to acid (such as misoprostol), even if I also chose to use one of the new COX-2 drugs. And people with borderline kidney or heart function should probably not take any type of NSAID.

One consideration that may have been exaggerated is convenience. Some NSAIDs need to be taken four times daily, others twice daily and a small number once daily. For most people this is not important, but for others, especially if they're likely to forget a midday dose at work, it very definitely is.

The choice of the NSAIDs tried, and the order in which they are tried, is influenced by their safety profiles. More on that later.

Just how good are NSAIDs in arthritis?

Not as good as we would like. In the most common types of arthritis – rheumatoid arthritis (RA) and osteoarthritis (OA) – NSAIDs are certainly useful, but by themselves they are woefully inadequate.

With RA, common practice is to find the best NSAID and then decide on a second-line drug to be added. It is seldom that the disease is so mild as to be controlled by NSAIDs alone.

With OA there may be an inflammatory component that is helped by an NSAID, but the chief benefit seems to be pain control. Studies have found that, in OA, a simple analgesic such as paracetamol is often just as good as an NSAID, and safer and cheaper.

In some diseases NSAIDs are very effective: in crystal arthritis, such as gout, NSAID response is spectacular – unless treatment is started too late or the dose is inadequate. In ankylosing spondylitis, an NSAID usually results in the patient's first good night of sleep in years.

Side effects of the older NSAIDs

Common side effects

- indigestion,
- stomach ulceration and bleeding,

Rare side effects

- skin rash, including photosensitivity (a rash provoked by going out in the sun) and hives,
- jaundice or other evidence of liver problems,
- bowel ulceration and bleeding,
- impaired production of blood cells (aplastic anaemia),
- asthma,
- significant kidney impairment,
- confusion, headache and neck stiffness.

Some of the rarer side effects are linked to specific NSAIDs (such as aplastic anaemia with phenylbutazone), whilst others may be seen with any NSAID. For example, if an asthma attack is provoked by one NSAID, all (including aspirin) should be avoided. In special circumstances, if the NSAID is badly needed, the patient can be desensitised.

All NSAIDs also seem to affect kidney blood flow. This is not a problem for most people, but it's a big problem for:

- older people,

- people with kidney function that is already below normal,

- people taking some other drugs (such as diuretics, given to get rid of excess body fluid or to treat high blood pressure).

These people may be affected quite badly, by worsening kidney function, more fluid retention, worsening blood pressure control and even heart failure.

The common side effects, those affecting the gut, are the real problem. NSAID indigestion is common; about 10–20 per cent of users will experience it at some time. But it's an unreliable marker for an ulcer, which can bleed without any warning signs. And many with indigestion don't have ulcers.

Taking an NSAID increases the risk of developing an ulcer, having gastrointestinal bleeding or experiencing an ulcer perforation by about five times. The risk of a bleeding ulcer in an otherwise healthy person taking one of the older NSAIDs has been estimated at 1 to 2 for every 100 'patient years'. In other words, if 100 patients take the NSAID for a year, 1 or 2 of them will develop an ulcer in that year.

Only about half of all ulcers will cause symptoms. Very often the first sign of an ulcer is evidence of bleeding, such as vomiting of blood, black bowel movements or light-headedness and fainting.

There are a number of ulcer-protective drugs available but only misoprostol and omeprazole have been convincingly shown to reduce the risk.

For indigestion alone, anti-ulcer drugs can be tried. They may or may not clear up the symptom. Because the cause of non-ulcer indigestion isn't known, it can be difficult to deal with. Sometimes it's so bad that the best solution is simply to stop the NSAID.

Other NSAID issues

Taking an NSAID on an 'as needed' basis (a pill or two today, then a few days skipped) is foolish. NSAIDs need several days to develop their full effect, and little can be expected from occasional doses except possibly heartburn or an ulcer. The ulcer doctors see much more ulcer bleeding in people who use NSAIDs only occasionally than they do in patients with arthritis. It's surprising how many people take aspirin for stomach aches or insomnia.

Most pharmacists recommend that an NSAID be taken with food. It's doubtful this really helps prevent an ulcer, but meals do help as reminders.

NSAIDs come in suppository form as well as tablets and capsules, but there's no evidence that suppositories cause fewer ulcers.

NSAIDs may interact with other drugs, and can cause real problems:

- with blood-thinning agents (anticoagulants), serious bleeding may result;

- with lithium, toxic blood levels of lithium can occur;

- with a variety of blood pressure medications, high blood pressure control may worsen; sulindac may possibly be the safest NSAID in this setting.

Finally, there is nothing magic about an NSAID. If you don't think it's helping, stop taking it. If symptoms of pain or stiffness or even increased joint swelling reappear, you need it and you can restart it. You may have to wait a few days to feel its full effect, but if it was helping before and nothing else has changed, it will work again.

Cortisone – the adrenocorticosteroids

Adrenocorticosteroids (also called corticosteroids) are the most powerful anti-inflammatory drugs we have. Were it not for their side effects we would use them much more freely. They are essential in the treatment of some forms of arthritis, such as SLE and polymyalgia rheumatica, where the decision to use them is taken with full knowledge of the risks involved. They are also widely used, in relatively low doses, in RA, where it is increasingly recognised that they may help prevent joint damage.

It was in RA that the first corticosteroid, cortisone, was used. In 1949, Dr Philip Hench of the Mayo Clinic gave it to a number of patients. The effect was spectacular. I've seen the 'before and after' movies Hench took of his patients, painfully climbing, and then leaping, over a bench barrier. So impressive was the result that Hench was among the winners of the 1950 Nobel prize in medicine. It was several years before it was realised that this 'cure' for RA was flawed and that it carried a price. That price was the syndrome of hypercortisonism.

First, though, a few words of clarification. There are a number of chemical compounds that qualify as 'steroids' – vitamin D and male sex hormones among them – but when the term is used in medicine it almost always refers to cortisol, produced by the adrenal gland, or one of its synthetic cousins. Of these, cortisone and hydrocortisone were the first to be made commercially; nowadays the most commonly used (and cheapest) is prednisone.

Problems with corticosteroids are of two types – those arising from using doses higher than the amount the body normally makes each day (the equivalent of about 7.5 milligrams of prednisone), and those arising from the sudden withdrawal of corticosteroid medication. The likelihood, and severity, of both are directly related to the size of the daily dose and the length of time it is taken.

Problems from high, and prolonged, corticosteroid use

Hypercortisonism

When the dose of prednisone (or another similar synthetic corticosteroid) exceeds 7.5 milligrams a day for more than three to four weeks, signs of hypercortisonism begin to develop. Hypercortisonism caused by prednisone is identical to Cushing's syndrome, a disease state where the adrenal glands produce too much cortisol.

Fully developed, hypercortisonism may include any or all of the following features:

- increased appetite and weight gain, especially on the trunk and face (a chubby face is typical of someone on high-dose, long-term prednisone);

- easy bruising and skin fragility of the arms and legs, especially in older people;

- cataract development;

- mood changes: mild euphoria is common, but depression may occur; insomnia is frequent;

- high blood pressure;

- extra insulin required by diabetics because of higher blood sugars, and 'pre-diabetics' becoming overtly diabetic;

- stomach ulcers, if the patient is taking NSAIDs at the same time;

- stunting of growth in children.

Osteonecrosis

'Osteonecrosis' is doctor-talk for dead bone. It is a specific type of dead bone, the kind that results when an area of bone loses its blood supply. If this happens near a joint – and the hip is a favourite target – the area of dead bone may collapse, a catastrophe that inevitably ends up with surgery and a total hip replacement.

Cortisone-like drugs have for a long time been seen as the culprit in osteonecrosis, although this has been hard to prove. Many diseases for which corticosteroids are used – such as SLE and Crohn's disease – may themselves be responsible for osteonecrosis.

Fortunately, osteonecrosis from prednisone is rare. I've never yet had a patient develop it.

Hardening of the arteries (atherosclerosis)

There is no question that the long-term use of prednisone in systemic lupus erythematosus increases the risk of hardening of the arteries and, in particular, coronary artery disease. These conditions substantially increase the risk of stroke and heart attack. There is still some debate as to whether prednisone has the same effect in RA. Antimalarial drugs, such as hydroxychloroquine, have an opposite, protective effect. Because they are also helpful in treating the inflammation of both diseases, this 'side effect' is a real bonus and can justify treatment with these two drugs at the same time.

Osteoporosis

Bone is a living tissue. Old bone is continuously being broken down, in patches. This process is followed almost immediately by the laying down of new bone by bone-forming cells. The two processes of breakdown and repair are normally in balance. When the rate of breakdown exceeds repair, bone mass (solidity) is reduced. We call this osteoporosis.

Between 10 and 20 per cent of all patients with RA, who are on long-term corticosteroids, will experience crush fractures of one or more vertebrae in the backbone. The risk of hip fracture is 50 per cent.

This risk of fracture can be estimated in any patient, taking corticosteroids or not, by measuring bone mineral density (through a technique known as DEXA – dual energy X-ray absorptiometry). Ordinary X-rays won't do; up to half of bone mass must be lost before they will detect the change.

How does osteoporosis come about?

Bone breakdown continues at a constant rate throughout life. The rate of bone repair, however, slows down in older people. It also slows in those who are physically inactive, in post-menopausal women with the drop in oestrogen production, and in those who get inadequate supplies of calcium and vitamin D (see Figure 7.1). Often, many of these factors are combined.

Corticosteroids magnify problems in bone repair. They can cause osteoporosis in anyone, young or old, but the effect is most obvious in post-menopausal women (who already have many of the osteoporosis risk factors). They do this quite quickly, particularly within the first 6 to 12 months of treatment. Corticosteroids affect several key elements in bone repair. The amount of calcium available for new bone formation is reduced. Cortico-steroids both slow dietary calcium absorption in the intestine and speed its removal from blood by the kidney. They stimulate the bone cells that promote bone breakdown, and inhibit the bone cells that promote bone growth.

What this means is that every patient who is started on prednisone for anything but a very short period must also be started on an anti-osteoporosis programme.

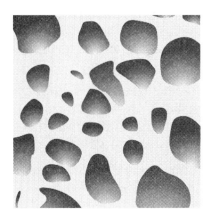 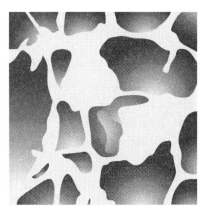

Figure 7.1 Normal versus osteoporotic bone. The picture on the left shows a cross-section of a normal vertebra; that on the right shows the effects of osteoporotic depletion.

Your risk of osteoporosis is also increased if

- You are a post-menopausal woman
- Your menstrual periods started late (after 14) or ended early (before 40)
- You are white or Asian
- You are housebound and elderly
- You weigh less than 55 kg (120 pounds)
- You smoke cigarettes

- In the past I often recommended oestrogen treatment if the patient was a post-menopausal woman. Now that I know of the risks of heart disease and cancer with oestrogen, I don't do this.

- A regular programme of aerobic physical activity should be designed, if necessary with the assistance of a physiotherapist, keeping in mind the problems imposed by the arthritis.

- A daily calcium intake of at least 1,000 milligrams should be achieved. One cup of milk will provide 300 milligrams, a cup of yogurt about 400 milligrams. Calcium-containing antacid tablets are another inexpensive source.

- A low dose (1,000 units) of vitamin D daily is desirable. Vitamin D is essential to normal bone development. People who are elderly or housebound are very often deficient in vitamin D, and have a greatly increased risk of fracture.

- If I expect that the patient will need more than 5 milligrams of prednisone for more than three months, I will also prescribe one of the bisphosphonates – etidronate (the weakest), alendronate or (if the patient already has osteoporosis and hasn't responded to treatment) pamidronate. Bisphosphonates are effective in both the treatment and prevention of osteoporosis.

Problems from the sudden withdrawal of corticosteroid medication

When corticosteroids are used in doses of more than the equivalent of 7.5 milligrams of prednisone a day, the adrenal gland does not make cortisol. This is not a problem if drugs such as prednisone are used for short periods only. But when such doses are used continuously for prolonged periods (three months is considered the cut-off), cortisol production will be completely suppressed. The patient is now dependent on a source outside the body for corticosteroid.

Because corticosteroids are essential for life, and are particularly important in helping the body deal with major physical stress, their sudden absence – if for any reason the patient stops taking daily prednisone – can have serious consequences. If adrenal gland suppression is only partial, symptoms of fatigue, nausea, loss of appetite and muscle pain may develop. If suppression is total, the patient may experience the life-threatening state doctors call 'shock'. The only safe way to reduce, and stop, corticosteroids is very slowly, over a period of weeks to months. But even if the patient has managed to achieve this, the body may not completely recover its ability to produce large amounts of cortisol in circumstances of stress until a year or more goes by.

Because of this, patients who are on (or have been on) corticosteroids must be given extra corticosteroid if they are exposed to severe physical stress. Such events as an automobile accident or major surgery call for immediate corticosteroid treatment, usually by needle, into a vein.

Patients taking corticosteroids should never stop their medication suddenly. If unable to take their regular dose, they should contact a doctor. They should also carry a wallet card (or wear a medical-alert bracelet) indicating that they are on a corticosteroid.

To sum up

The most effective way to avoid the unwelcome side effects of corticosteroids is not to take them. Regrettably, this is not always possible. Next best is to minimise the damage by attempting to keep the dose as low as possible most of the time, and to keep short any periods of high-dose treatment. If at all possible, the daily dose should be taken as a single morning dose, as normal cortisol production is much less likely to be suppressed when this is done. And corticosteroids should never be stopped suddenly if they have been taken continuously for more than a week or two.

'Second-line' drugs

The name 'second-line' comes from the fact that in RA the NSAIDs are used first. When their effect has been determined, assuming there is still a problem, the drugs in this next class are then called upon.

We used to call second-line drugs 'remitting agents', but it's clear that they don't cause the disease to go away. Some doctors call them DMARDs (disease-modifying anti-rheumatic drugs), which they are, and some call them SAARDs (slow-acting anti-rheumatic drugs), which they also are.

The two major differences, in practical terms, between these drugs and NSAIDs are that they take much longer to have an effect (usually months), and they are much more effective in suppressing the disease process. Unfortunately, another characteristic of drugs in this category is the fact that they often lose their effect as time goes by.

This means that, after several years, many patients will have acquired experience with quite a number of these agents. Fortunately, research into new drugs in this area has managed to keep pace. The list keeps getting longer, but the main second-line drugs at present are:

- methotrexate

- gold by injection

- azathioprine

- sulfasalazine

- hydroxychloroquine

- oral gold

These drugs are unrelated to each other chemically. Almost all were first used in arthritis for reasons that were later shown to be wrong, or as a result of a series of chance observations.

Gold, for instance, was used because RA was once thought to be caused by tuberculosis, and gold salts have some activity against TB in a test-tube. Methotrexate, when it was first used in psoriasis, was observed to help control psoriatic arthritis, so it was used in RA, where it was found to work even better. It is only now, in the age of genetic engineering, that we may be developing a series of 'designer drugs' specifically for arthritis.

When are these drugs used?

In rheumatoid arthritis, right away.

In a recent Dutch study, X-rays of 25 per cent of a group of patients who had experienced symptoms of RA for only three months showed signs of joint damage. A slightly older study compared a group of patients given a relatively weak drug (hydroxychloroquine) with a similar group given a placebo – something that today would be considered unethical. The placebo group, who were eventually (nine months later) put on effective treatment, never did catch up. Even after three years they had higher levels of pain and disability than those who were treated early.

Not only are these drugs more effective than NSAIDs alone in RA, I believe that almost all of them are much safer.

'Second-line drugs' were – and still are – primarily for the treatment of RA. They are used as well in psoriatic arthritis, although all too often they are only somewhat effective – or ineffective. Some of these drugs are used as 'supportive' treatment in a few other conditions, in particular ankylosing spondylitis, systemic lupus erythematosus, polymyositis and dermatomyositis. There is no 'second-line' treatment available for the most common problem of all, OA. Nor is there specific treatment for fibromyalgia, chondrocalcinosis, polymyalgia rheumatica, scleroderma or Sjögren's syndrome.

Which one to choose?

These are my preferred second-line drugs, in order of *safety*:

- hydroxychloroquine
- sulfasalazine
- methotrexate
- azathioprine
- sodium aurothiomalate – a gold compound given by intramuscular injection
- leflunomide
- ciclosporin

In order of *effectiveness*, my list looks like this:

- methotrexate
- sodium aurothiomalate
- leflunomide
- azathioprine
- hydroxychloroquine

I have dropped from my list a gold preparation that is taken by mouth (auranofin) because it is the least effective of the lot, and for a similar reason rarely use minocycline (an antibiotic that is modestly helpful in RA). Penicillamine I now no longer use because of its serious side effects.

Second-line drug combinations

One very exciting development in the past few years is the discovery that second-line drugs may be more effective when used in combination rather than singly. Some arthritis specialists start off with 'triple therapy' (methotrexate + sulfasalizine + hydroxychloroquine, plus or minus a course of prednisone) while others – like me – prefer to see what their preferred single agent (methotrexate) will do before deciding to double or triple up. I know, however, that whatever I decide to do, I have only a very short time to settle things down before permanent joint damage begins to develop.

Several proved effective combinations include:

- methotrexate and sulfasalizine and hydroxychloroquine
- methotrexate and leflunomide
- methotrexate and intramuscular gold
- methotrexate and ciclosporin
- methotrexate and infliximab
- methotrexate and etanercept

Leflunomide, infliximab and etanercept are part of the 'new wave' of second-line drugs (see below)

Methotrexate (MTX)

Unless a patient has very mild rheumatoid arthritis (then I might prescribe hydroxychloroquine), this is my first choice. It works fairly quickly, it works for most, and it continues to be effective for a longer period than almost all other second-line drugs. It is also – despite the very frightening list of possible side effects – one of the safest drugs I use. I also use it in psoriatic arthritis and

occasionally (particularly if I am trying to lower the dose of prednisone the patient needs) in SLE and polymyositis.

Methotrexate is different from most drugs in that it is given
just once a week – on the same day each week. It is usually taken
in pill form, all the pills together at one time, but in about 10 to 15
per cent of patients, nausea (on the 'pill' day or the next day) is a
problem. Then I prescribe it in injectable form (and arrange for a
nurse to teach the patient how to do this – subcutaneously, just
like diabetics self-inject with insulin).

The dose range of weekly methotrexate varies from two to ten
2.5-milligram tablets, and my current practice is to raise the
weekly dose fairly quickly – over two to three months – until the
symptoms and signs of arthritis are completely suppressed. If this
doesn't happen within that time period, I start to consider adding
in one or more other 'second-line' drugs. Time is really very
important in preventing long-term damage.

Side effects of methotrexate

Note that impairment of kidney function increases the risk of any
of these side effects. NSAIDs don't interact with MTX when
MTX is taken in the doses recommended; however, sulfa-
containing antibiotics increase the risk of side effects and should
be avoided. Side effects are often dealt with by decreasing the
dose or temporarily stopping MTX and then restarting it.

Common to occasional

- A 12- to 24-hour reaction to the weekly dose, in the form of
  nausea or profound fatigue.

- Mild anaemia, and occasionally lower numbers of white
  blood cells or platelets; a complete blood count (and blood
  tests for liver damage) should be done every two weeks at the
  beginning, then monthly and later every six to eight weeks.

- Small sores inside the mouth; these may be prevented by
  taking 1 milligram of folic acid (a vitamin that can be
  purchased without a prescription) every day.

- A small amount of hair loss, noticeable on the pillow each
  morning but not obvious to friends and neighbours.

- Temporary reduction in the sperm count in men may be caused by MTX. In women, MTX should be avoided in pregnancy (it can cause a miscarriage) and breast-feeding.

Rare (if you suspect one of these, stop MTX and call your doctor)

- Significant lowering of blood counts (haemoglobin, white blood cells, platelets) with symptoms of tiredness, dizziness, infection, bruising or bleeding.

- Cramps and diarrhea.

- 'Allergic pneumonia' – fever, cough that doesn't bring up anything, shortness of breath.

- Infection, including pneumonia and shingles.

- Skin rash (very uncommon). Occasionally, patients with RA who have rheumatoid nodules will develop many new ones, even though the arthritis is under good control.

Very rare

- Liver damage. To be on the safe side, no use of alcohol (except at weddings, birthdays and Christmas), because alcohol may combine with MTX to damage the liver. Psoriasis, obesity and possibly diabetes may also increase the risk of MTX liver damage.

Possible but not proved

- A very few cases of lymphoma (a type of lymph gland cancer) have been discovered in patients treated with MTX (see below under 'Azathioprine'). These resolved when MTX was stopped.

Sodium aurothiomalate (gold by injection)

Intramuscular gold is the traditional number 1 drug in RA, with over 50 years of clinical use. There is little risk of an unexpected surprise with gold, and it has a reasonably sustained effect over the long term. The major disadvantages include the need to visit the doctor each week, and the long time it may take to begin to work (12 to 20 weeks).

To make sure the patient isn't sensitive to gold, two small test doses of aurothiomalate are given, one week apart. After that, the regular dose (50 milligrams) is given once a week. The practice in the past was to do this, once a week, until 1,000 milligrams had been given, and some doctors still do this. If the patient is no better, they then try another drug. The problem is that some patients may show a great deal of improvement long before five months (the time needed to give 1,000 milligrams) are up and others will need quite a bit longer.

Most rheumatologists will start to space the doses out, at first to every second week, and then to every third, when they feel the maximum benefit has been reached. It's possible, but unusual, to be able to space the doses out to once a month. Once a patient is on a 'maintenance schedule', it is continued indefinitely (for years), even if the arthritis seems to have disappeared. If the arthritis flares up (it very often does), it is important to realise that the gold hasn't lost its effect. It simply needs to be given more often.

Because the side effects involving the blood and urine may turn up at any time, the patient should have a blood and urine test each time an injection is given, although if the patient has been safely on gold for several years, this is sometimes spaced out to every second injection.

Side effects of gold injections

Common to occasional

- Sore mouth and itchy skin, often the first sign of side effects. If gold is continued on the same schedule, mouth ulceration and more extensive skin rash may result. The dose should be withheld for a week or two, until the symptoms subside. Injections can then be resumed, either with a reduced dose or with an increased interval between shots.

Rare

- Flare-up of arthritis symptoms, or facial 'flushing' and headache, following the weekly injection. This is often controlled by the use of prednisone, given only on the day of the injection. There is no risk of steroid side effects with this.

- Thrombocytopenia (a drop in the level of platelets in the blood). If this level falls below a certain point, there is a risk of bruising or even uncontrolled bleeding. The drop is due to an allergic reaction to the gold, and most often reverses if the drug is stopped. Sometimes steroids are used to treat the allergic reaction and speed recovery.

- Proteinuria (the 'leakage' of a protein [albumin] into the urine in abnormally high amounts). Normally the kidney filter is very fine, but an allergic reaction to gold may cause the kidney 'pores' to enlarge and allow the large albumin molecules to escape. Proteinuria is very much like thrombocytopenia. It clears up when gold is stopped, but this may take some time and may require corticosteroids.

Very rare

- A drop in the white blood cell count, or aplastic anaemia (where the bone marrow stops production of red and white blood cells, as well as platelets). These complications may be fatal.

- Colitis, with severe diarrhoea.

- Hepatitis.

- Gold 'pneumonia' (lung inflammation due to drug hyper-sensitivity).

- Severe generalised skin rash.

Azathioprine

Over the last few years I have found myself using more and more of this agent for RA, primarily in instances where methotrexate and gold have failed. It is also used for systemic lupus erythe-matosus and in some people with psoriatic arthritis. It's a fairly safe and effective drug that usually begins to give relief after two to three months, and continues to work moderately well over the long term.

Azathioprine is taken daily. The initial dose is one tablet (50 milligrams), and the dose is later adjusted according to the person's weight. Later, if the patient has done well, the dose can often be reduced without losing the effect. Once a regular dose has been settled on, complete blood counts and liver tests are needed less frequently than with methotrexate and gold, but still should be checked at least every three months.

Side effects of azathioprine

Common to occasional

- Mild nausea

- Fatigue

- Fever

Rare

- Hepatitis, with fever, skin rash and liver-enzyme abnormalities.

- Low haemoglobin, low white blood cell count (and possible infection).

- Skin rash.

Very rare or possible but not proved

- Malignant lymphoma. Experience in kidney transplant patients has led to concern, and long-standing debate, as to whether azathioprine can cause this type of lymph gland cancer in people with RA.

Even without azathioprine, the risk of lymphoma for people with RA is increased slightly over the risk in the general population. One study has suggested that azathioprine doubles this extremely small risk. On the other hand, a long-term British study of patients receiving azathioprine for inflammatory bowel disease failed to demonstrate any increase in cancer risk. There were no patients with lymphoma reported.

Sulfasalazine

North American experience with this drug in the treatment of RA has been limited, but because it's a mainstay in the treatment of inflammatory bowel disease, its side effects are well known. Britain seems to be quite enthusiastic, and to rank it somewhere near intramuscular gold. Its safety profile is very encouraging, it's fairly effective, and it takes action in two to three months. Its benefits are sustained moderately well over the long term.

There are conflicting reports as to whether sulfasalazine is useful in some of the seronegative arthritis conditions, particularly psoriatic arthritis and ankylosing spondylitis.

Sulfasalazine should be started with a low dose and gradually built up. It starts with one tablet (500 milligrams) a day for a week, then the daily dose is increased by one tablet each week until, by the fourth week, the patient is taking two tablets twice a day. Occasionally the dose is increased to three tablets twice a day. Once a final dose has been settled on, complete blood counts and liver tests are done monthly.

Side effects of sulfasalazine

Warning – this drug contains sulfa and should not be taken if you are allergic to sulfa drugs.

Common to occasional

- Nausea or vague abdominal 'unease'.
- Loss of appetite.
- 'Dizziness', headache.
- Temporary lowering of the sperm count in men (reversible when the drug is stopped).
- Yellowish-orange discoloration of the urine.

Rare

- Skin rash, which may be quite extensive and severe.

Very rare

- Severe drop in white blood cell count and platelet count, with infection and bleeding (from the gut, the kidneys, the skin, mucus membranes, etc.) possible.

- 'Allergic' hepatitis (due to drug hypersensitivity).

- 'Allergic' pneumonia (due to drug hypersensitivity.

Penicillamine

The dose of this drug has to be built up very slowly to avoid very serious (though rare) side effects. Nevertheless, when other drugs fail, penicillamine may be used because it helps many. It begins to give relief within three to six months, and the effects continue moderately well over the long term.

It's important to start with a low daily dose of penicillamine (no more than 250 milligrams), and only slowly increase the daily dose (125–250 milligrams each time, no more often than every eight weeks). The maximum daily dose should not exceed 1,000 milligrams. Penicillamine should be taken on an empty stomach, no closer to a meal than one hour, or it won't all be absorbed into the body.

Despite its name, this drug does not cross-react with penicillin. People with penicillin allergy may take it.

Side effects of penicillamine

Common to occasional

- Mild nausea, metallic taste in the mouth.

- Minor skin rash, sores in the mouth.

- Small amounts of protein in the urine.

Rare

- Drop in platelet count (with risk of bleeding).

- Large amounts of protein in the urine (see under 'Side effects of gold injection', above).

Very rare

- Can cause illnesses that look like dermatomyositis, systemic lupus erythematosus or myasthenia gravis (a condition of severe muscle weakness).

- Major drop in red cell, white blood cell count

Hydroxychloroquine

Hydroxychloroquine is a drug originally developed for use against malaria, but it has been found to be very helpful in several kinds of arthritis. It's considered to be much weaker than almost all the other 'slow-acting drugs'. Its safety profile, however, is so good that in someone with relatively mild RA it's a good choice. It takes effect in three to six months, but its long-term benefit in RA is not as good as that of other drugs.

It's also used in systemic lupus erythematosus, particularly if skin, joint and muscle symptoms are prominent. It seems to counteract the effect of raising the amount of lipid (blood-fat) caused by the corticosteroids that are often used in these same patients. Occasionally it's very helpful in psoriatic arthritis, although in a few patients the psoriasis will worsen significantly.

It's very important, if the risk of eye damage (see the section on side effects, below) is to be avoided, that, in addition to annual eye checks, the dose is carefully calculated, based on the person's 'ideal' body weight. The maximum daily dose is 400 milligrams of hydroxychloroquine (200 milligrams twice a day), but that is for anyone over 59 kg (130 pounds). Those who weigh less must take less. Someone weighing 50 kg (110 pounds) should get 300 milligrams daily. Using these precautions, I have never seen or heard of a patient developing eye damage.

Side effects of hydroxychloroquine

Common to occasional

- Nausea, mild abdominal discomfort.

Rare

- Skin rash.

- Muscle weakness.

- Dizziness.

Very rare

- Permanent damage to the retina of the eye, leading to blindness. Fewer than a dozen cases of this have been reported in the world medical literature in patients for whom hydroxychloroquine (as opposed to the older drug chloroquine) was used, where kidney function was normal and the dose was based on body weight. Nevertheless, an annual eye check is prudent.

Auranofin

Gold by mouth has proved to be a disappointment. Initially it was hoped it would be as effective as gold given by intramuscular injection. However, it isn't, and with its annoying tendency to cause diarrhoea it has slipped to last place on most physicians' lists. It has a good safety record but doesn't take effect until after three to four months, and the long-term benefits are below average.

There is very little flexibility in the dose of auranofin – one 3-milligram tablet twice a day. A complete blood count and urinalysis should be done monthly.

Side effects of auranofin

Common to occasional

- Abdominal discomfort, loose stools, diarrhoea.

- Skin rash.

Very rare

- Protein in urine.

- Lowered blood count.

Ciclosporin

Introduced as a means of blocking the rejection of organ transplants (such as kidney grafts), this powerful immuno-suppressive has been quite effective in RA. There are some real advantages in combining it with methotrexate: the effect may be better than the effect of either drug used alone, and a lower dose of ciclosporin can be used. A lower dose reduces the risk of side effects.

I don't use the combination often. I usually reserve it for cases in which methotrexate in full doses has failed to 'put out the fire' and I am very concerned that joint damage will occur in the immediate future.

The daily dose is calculated on ideal body weight. It can be taken with food, but never with grapefruit juice, which can increase the amount of drug your body absorbs and lead to side effects. A number of drugs can also affect the level of ciclosporin in your body: some antibiotics, antifungal agents, anticonvulsants and even some heart and blood pressure medicines. Check with your doctor or pharmacist if you are on any of these.

Because ciclosporin can cause high blood pressure and affect kidney function, blood pressure and kidney blood tests should be checked carefully before treatment and every two weeks for the first three months, then once a month.

Side effects of ciclosporin

- Rise in serum creatinine (indicating reduced kidney function).
- Raised blood pressure.
- Headache.
- Nausea.
- Increase in body hair.
- Fluid retention (ankle swelling).
- Hand tremor (shakiness).

Depending on the nature of the side effect, I either reduce the daily dose or stop the ciclosporin entirely. Fortunately, this has been necessary in only a few of my patients.

There is no convincing evidence that ciclosporin increases the risk of infection or cancer. However, it should not be used if there is an existing cancer or infection, just as it should not be used in people with abnormal kidney function or uncontrolled high blood pressure.

The new 'biologicals' – etanercept, infliximab, anakinra and adaluminab

These are the 'new kids on the block'. They were specifically designed to affect rheumatoid inflammation.

Inflammation in RA is a very complex process. We believe it starts when one of the class of cells that guards the body against foreign invaders (in ordinary inflammation these are usually bacteria or viruses) comes into contact with something that triggers the alarm. One form the alarm takes is a whole battery of chemical messengers, called cytokines, that are released into the joint. These recruit other cells, the white blood cells that produce antibodies and the white blood cells that attack and kill other cells and bacteria. One form this killing takes is the release into the immediate area of very 'corrosive' chemicals. Joint tissue, an innocent bystander, is damaged. Furthermore, cytokines stimulate the lining of the joint to grow and produce other chemicals that break down cartilage. Cytokines are released into the blood stream, and cause fever and fatigue. Finally, because the body is so finely balanced, there are also cytokines released that tend to damp down the inflammation. Unfortunately, in the joint affected by RA these 'good' cytokines tend to become overwhelmed by the 'bad' or pro-inflammatory cytokines.

One of the key cytokines that promotes inflammation is a substance called TNF-alpha. Produced by both the 'guard' cells (macrophages) and the joint-lining tissues, it is released into the surrounding tissues, joint fluid and blood. It stimulates other white blood cells to expand the inflammatory reaction. To do this it must attach itself to the other cells at a specific binding site – like a key in a lock.

Etanercept and infliximab have been designed to interfere

with this stimulatory action of TNF-alpha. *Etanercept* does this very cleverly; it's a molecule that looks exactly like the 'keyhole'. As long as there is enough of it in circulation (you have to inject it twice weekly under the skin), it will prevent enough 'keys' from finding the 'lock' they were intended for, and the inflammation will be damped down.

Infliximab has a similar effect, but it consists of an antibody (a protein specifically designed to attach to another protein) against TNF-alpha. Once the 'key' has an antibody stuck to it, it no longer fits the 'lock'. Infliximab too has to be given by injection – in this case into a vein – but fortunately only once every two months.

Experience with both infliximab and etanercept has reminded us that there is a 'good' side to inflammation as well as a bad side. By damping down the inflammatory response we also damp down the body's ability to deal with infections. This means that the use of the drugs must be suspended if any infection – such as in the bladder or kidney, sinus or lung, or even skin – occurs, and until it is dealt with. Otherwise, the infection may get out of hand and cause serious harm. Fortunately, this is not often a problem.

An even more serious, even if uncommon, infection has been associated with infliximab: the activation of 'latent' tuberculosis. In practice, this means that all my patients who are started on either drug get a TB skin test and a chest X-ray first; if there is a suggestion of 'hidden' TB, they get TB treatment in addition to their arthritis drugs.

These new drugs are not always as effective as we had initially hoped, but they do help many people whose RA has not been controlled with the older 'second-line' drugs. In addition, we have discovered that they may be extremely effective in the spondarthropathies – psoriatic arthritis and ankylosing spondylitis. Because, up to now, we have had very little to offer individuals with those conditions, these drugs represent a real breakthrough.

The big drawback of these new treatments is their price – considerably more than the older standbys. My feeling is that, if they prevent joint damage and disability, they will pay for themselves many times over. I expect that in a few years most people with RA will be given a reasonable but short time on methotrexate, and if they don't improve, one of these newcomers will be added. Already there are other 'newcomers' – another antibody against TNF (*adaluminab*) and a drug that blocks another cytokine, IL-1 (*anakinra*). There are many more in development, all designed to target (and block) individual steps in the very complex 'falling domino' sequence that leads to joint inflammation.

And even more new drugs, here and on the horizon

In addition to focusing on drugs that block inflammation, research scientists have worked to develop other drugs that 'blunt' the immune cells that play a key role in rheumatoid inflammation.

Leflunomide is one such drug, which acts on a key cell called a lymphocyte. It is clearly helpful in RA, and early research shows that it has promise in psoriatic arthritis and systemic lupus erythematosus. I use it in combination with methotrexate in patients whose RA is difficult to control; only if these two drugs fail do I consider the more expensive etanercept or infliximab. Diarrhoea (particularly if the higher doses originally recommended are used) and high blood pressure are two side effects to watch for, and I get the same set of monitoring blood tests I order for methotrexate. Liver test abnormalities and low white blood counts are the things I am looking out for.

Another drug, *rituximab*, is designed to target a specific type of B-lymphocyte. Originally used to treat a form of B-cell cancer, it has now been shown to be effective in RA as well as in a variety of other auto-immune disorders. I have no experience with this drug so far, and suspect it will be used only if and when the very rare patient has failed to respond to my usual treatment.

Minocycline

A popular North American radio doctor has for several years pushed the use of tetracycline-group antibiotics for just about every kind of arthritis and muscle ache and pain. His reasoning is that there are all sorts of infectious organisms in people, and that infectious organisms have been shown to trigger certain kinds of arthritis. Besides, he reasons, tetracycline-group antibiotics – including minocycline and doxycycline – can't hurt. So, many of my patients ask me for antibiotics for their arthritis. I tell them that:

- Life is a lot more complicated than that. Although infection may play a role in some kinds of arthritis, it has not been proven in most. It is a very old idea – 60 years ago, doctors recommended that people with RA undergo total dental extraction and sinus drainage surgery on the theory that the arthritis was caused by chronic infection.

- Minocycline does more than kill bugs. It also interferes with the release of a chemical (nitric oxide) that kills cartilage cells and with enzymes that break down cartilage. It may do other good things, such as interfere with inflammation and immune reactions.

- Research has shown that minocycline, taken for several months, is helpful – especially in mild, early RA. I think it is about as effective as hydroxychloroquine or auranofin. I certainly would not recommend it as a single, first-choice drug to anyone with aggressive RA.

- Minocycline may be worth a try in combination with another second-line drug – when methotrexate has been helpful, for instance, but there is still a fair amount of inflammation.

Side effects of minocycline

Most side effects are mild – although dizziness, nausea and headache may cause up to a quarter of patients to abandon the drug. There have also been a very few instances when, used to treat acne, minocycline caused systemic lupus erythematosus and autoimmune hepatitis. And hyperpigmentation of the skin or gums – blue-grey discoloration either diffusely in the skin and gums, or locally, in old skin scars – is fairly common. Both types gradually fade when minocycline is stopped.

Physiotherapy, occupational therapy and social services

The following illustrates how my community's arthritis treatment team works here in Canada. Obviously the situation varies from country to country, but I offer this as an example of what may happen.

Debbie is a 33-year-old primary school teacher. She and her husband Mike have been married for three years.

Debbie came to me because of progressive joint pain and swelling over the past year. Despite her pain, and the severe fatigue that accompanied it, I sensed that she probably wouldn't have come if she weren't having trouble coping at work — she'd been forced to take a total of ten sick days over the past four months.

My diagnosis was rheumatoid arthritis and, after an initial period of NSAID treatment alone, I started Debbie on methotrexate and low-dose prednisone.

Debbie was obviously relieved that I could put a label on her problem. She had been concerned that her symptoms were 'all in her head', and suspected that Mike thought so, too. This relief, though, was short-lived. She began to push herself harder. She took on extra responsibilities at school and spent her weekends trying to ensure that her home was immaculate. She tried to deal with her illness by denying its existence.

This phase didn't last. On a visit a month or two after the diagnosis had been made, she broke into tears. She confessed that she wasn't sleeping and had difficulty concentrating. She was depressed.

I realised that both Debbie and I needed help. I asked her if she would like to see our arthritis team's social worker. I explained that she could only benefit from an exploration of her emotional reactions to her arthritis. I also thought the social worker could help her develop more constructive strategies to deal with the realities of chronic illness. Debbie agreed, and I made the referral. And realising that in my focus on controlling her arthritis with drugs I had ignored other equally important aspects of treatment, I requested both a physiotherapy and an occupational therapy consultation.

The social worker comments

During our first session, I explained to Debbie that she would have an opportunity to explore the impact that arthritis had on her personally, on her relationships and on her place in the community. We agreed to meet for several sessions to do some problem-solving in the areas Debbie identified as stressors.

Individual intervention

Debbie confessed that her self-esteem had taken a beating. It had always been linked to her ability to demonstrate, to herself and to others, that she could take on a challenge. Her sense of worth, being tied to her productivity, had nose-dived.

In our discussions, Debbie came to realise that the message she received as she was growing up was 'the harder you work, the better', and that this was now working against her. She came to recognise that self-worth does not depend on accomplishments. What were important were her unique qualities as a person, her personality, her strengths and skills, and these arthritis could never take away from her.

She began to practise 'self-talk'. When a negative message, such as 'I feel useless, as I can't even clean my own home any more', cropped up, she learned to rephrase the statement. 'Even though there are some things I'm not able to do any more, there are many things I still can do.' As she practised this skill, Debbie's sense of self-worth gradually returned and she began to feel some control over her life again.

Reactions to her illness – shock, denial, frustration, anger – were explored. Debbie was pleased to discover that this was a normal, and necessary, process of adaptation.

Debbie also began to re-evaluate her priorities. She discovered that she had been preoccupied with the accumulation of material goods. She came to realise that this mattered little when placed against the importance of family and friends.

Marital intervention

Debbie and Mike had enjoyed a happy first few years of marriage, but since the onset of the arthritis both had felt increasingly distant from each other. Because Debbie was tired so much of the time, she and Mike spent much less time going out together, or even just talking. From Mike's perspective, Debbie seemed to have lost interest in him. Although she complained of pain, she looked well to him. The household tasks were no longer being done and Mike even caught himself wondering if she was getting lazy. He was also concerned about Debbie's reduced interest in sex, and, when they did make love, thoughts that he might be hurting her kept intruding. Debbie, on the other hand, began to feel that Mike wasn't being supportive. She was angry that he didn't help more around the house, and suspected he was worried about the financial consequences if she had to take a leave of absence from her job.

Debbie was relieved that Mike agreed to join us for a series of meetings. It didn't take long for both to realise that they had been experiencing their own emotional reactions to the arthritis, and that the first effect of this was that they were talking less and less to each other.

They began to make adjustments. Mike began to do the grocery shopping and some of the household tasks. They very tentatively learned to express clearly their feelings to each other. They learned to talk openly about their sexual relationship and how each of their needs might be met.

Mike also – and for the first time – went to Debbie's appointment with her rheumatologist, in an attempt to gain a better understanding of her arthritis.

Financial and vocational intervention

Debbie and Mike were worried that Debbie might not be able to continue working. They had just purchased a home and were concerned about meeting the mortgage payments on one salary. Resources such as short-term and long-term disability pensions, and vocational rehabilitation, were discussed as potential options. Fortunately for Debbie, she was able to continue teaching. She did make a few changes in her life. She obtained a special 'disabled person' parking permit, began to use a chair much more in the classroom, and hired someone to clean the house once a week.

I was pleased with the courage that Debbie and Mike demonstrated in coming to talk to me. I was also pleased that the result seemed to be good – a couple with revised and realistic priorities, with new strategies to cope with chronic illness, and with a relationship now based on honesty and openness. My guess is that they are now closer to each other than ever before.

Group intervention

To consolidate gains Debbie made in the individual and marital work, she was referred to a psychosocial group, in order to allow her to interact with others who have arthritis and who were coping with similar challenges.

The group consisted of eight sessions, and was professionally led. In exploring topics of common concern, Debbie found great relief in realising that she was not the only one who was experiencing difficulty in coping with credibility issues, loss of self-esteem and role changes, strong emotional reactions to the diagnosis, changes in her relationships and moodiness due to living with chronic pain. Following the group sessions, Debbie felt a renewed sense of motivation to meet the challenges of living with arthritis.

The physiotherapist comments

When Debbie was first seen, her morning stiffness didn't clear for two hours and she was fatigued all day long. Her hand grip strength was only a third of normal – not surprising in view of the fact that most of her finger joints, along with her left wrist, were swollen, and she was unable even to come close to making a tight fist. In addition to these joints, her shoulders and her foot MTP joints were painful with movement. Her shoulder movement was limited by about 20 per cent. Her left knee had a small amount of swelling, but a great deal of pain when she went up and down the stairs at school. In all, she had a total of 20 inflamed joints. She also had decreased strength in her thigh muscles. Neck pain, possibly related to poor posture at work, was an additional problem.

One part of Debbie's job was teaching physical education twice a week. She had always been proud of her physical fitness, but in the past year, because of her pain, stiffness and fatigue, her level of general activity was greatly reduced. It was evident she needed a generalised graded exercise programme to regain lost ground.

The problem of pain was partially addressed with the application of ice to all inflamed joints. Debbie purchased ice packs, including extras to use at work. She was shown how to apply them to painful joints, for 15 minutes each session, as frequently as needed. Initially, her left shoulder and left knee received most of this attention, but she also found that applying the pack direct to the soles of her feet gave relief.

I was concerned about the lack of movement in her left wrist and hands, and showed Debbie a general range-of-motion programme that involved all her joints, including her neck. I stressed the importance of working this programme into her daily schedule, repeating each exercise five times, twice a day. I told her that she might need to use ice applications before each session – and after, if necessary.

Dressing each morning took considerable time, but this (and the duration of her morning stiffness) was shortened considerably after she began starting the day with a hot shower and a run through her exercises.

For neck strain, Debbie was taught posture correction for sitting, standing and lying. She rehearsed this daily, and worked it into her normal activities to the point where she was correcting her posture a minimum of 25 times a day. The emphasis was on chin retraction and pelvic tilting, sitting and standing. An orthopaedic pillow was provided, and a special orthopaedic back support was recommended for when sitting. Debbie found it particularly helpful when driving and using the computer.

At this stage, with her arthritis far from being controlled, a delicate balance between activity and rest had to be maintained, and this was underlined. She already was well aware of the benefits of good physical fitness. I felt she would benefit from a pool (hydrotherapy) programme, and so referred her to one led by an experienced physiotherapist. It emphasised achieving a full range of movement of all joints and aimed at a moderate level of conditioning. Later, she progressed to swimming lengths at a neighbourhood pool. As her feet became less painful, she resumed her daily half-hour walks in proper footwear. I also told her about a local tai chi programme that could improve her overall fitness.

As important as all this was, Debbie needed a lot of information and a lot of reassurance. She had been given prescriptions for methotrexate, low-dose prednisone and naproxen. What she had read about the first two quite frankly frightened her, and she had put off getting the prescriptions filled. This isn't uncommon.

I gave her pamphlets on them, and discussed with her their benefits and side effects. The importance of regular blood checks, particularly with methotrexate, was stressed. Our information package on RA was also discussed with Debbie.

Two months later, after a total of six treatment sessions, Debbie was discharged from the active physiotherapy case load. I told her that the Arthritis Society would be available if there was a need in the future. She was doing extremely well. Morning stiffness was only 20 minutes, fatigue was delayed until after 3 p.m., and she no longer needed ice on a daily basis. Knees and feet were much better and, though a number of knuckles were still puffy, she had regained 95 per cent of her ability to make a fist. She was on a regular home programme of resisted isometric exercise for her shoulders and right knee, and was beginning to work on her left knee. (These exercises involve contracting the muscles without significant joint movement, usually done against resistance, such as pushing one's hands against each other.) Neck pain had settled down and she was able to sit at the computer for extended periods without problems. She was still involved in the pool programme, once a week, and was swimming on her own at the local swimming pool each weekend. Most important of all, she knew much more about her disease and the techniques required for a successful self-management programme.

The occupational therapist comments

My role included vocational intervention, modification of activities of daily living and, to a limited extent, marital intervention.

Vocational intervention
Debbie and I identified a number of problem areas at work. Her classroom was on the first floor of the school. Knee and foot pain and fatigue made negotiating stairs painful and difficult. In her classroom, she was experiencing problems raising her arm high enough to write on the blackboard, and gripping the chalk was a challenge. Her desk chair was hard, supported her back poorly and was without arm rests; every time she wanted to sit, she had to pull it out from the desk. Writing in her teacher's daily journal was difficult, as was pressing hard enough to make triplicate copies of report cards.

I met the head teacher and, eventually, his superior at the school board. It took some time to implement change but changes were made. These had a marked effect on Debbie's life.

Her classroom was relocated to the main floor, close to the staff room and washroom. The parking spot closest to her class was designated for her exclusive use. She switched to an overhead projector, reducing blackboard use, and when she did use the board she used only the bottom half and gripped the chalk with a special holder. She was given a higher chair to use while writing on overhead transparencies. Her new desk chair had appropriate back support, arm rests and could be adjusted for height. The computer setup was changed to reduce strain on her neck, shoulders and elbows while she was using it.

Physical education classes were rescheduled from 10 a.m. to 1 p.m., and Debbie had a 45-minute break at noon to rest. Two students, assigned in rotation each week, assisted with phys ed equipment setup and storage. Debbie switched from a briefcase to a backpack, reducing the stress on her hands and wrists, and she stopped wearing high heels to work.

Activities of daily living

Debbie and I identified quite a few problem areas. She had difficulty applying makeup, doing up small buttons, vacuuming and scrubbing the bathtub.

A large-handled blush applicator was suggested, and she switched from cream blush. A soft eyeliner was recommended. She discovered that a button hook was very helpful in fastening small buttons, particularly when morning stiffness added to her difficulties with dressing. An upright, lightweight vacuum replaced her heavy and awkward canister-style machine. She was encouraged to sit whenever possible when working in the kitchen. She and Mike are considering switching to lever-style handles on the kitchen and bathroom taps.

More than these details, the principles of energy conservation were reinforced – setting priorities, planning, pacing, using appropriate body mechanics and reorganising her working spaces.

Specific attention was paid to her hands and feet. Splints were made to support her wrists and reduce pain when they are being heavily stressed. Her right index finger had a flexion contracture – it was tight and was unable to straighten out. This interfered with the use of her hand. I made a splint, designed to stretch the finger out, for her to wear at night. It worked – every two weeks I could see improvement and remoulded the splint each time to accommodate the changes.

I taught Debbie to avoid hand activities that might contribute to hand deformities, and suggested she switch to a large-barrel pen, built-up utensils at home and lever-type door knobs and tap handles. I also checked to see that she was doing hand exercises to strengthen muscles and maintain movement.

To replace her high heels, I strongly recommended shoes with cushioning, a snug heel and adequate toe depth and width, and made sure she knew the name of a store where the staff was knowledgeable. Once she had these, I fitted them with customised insoles (foot orthotics).

Marital intervention

Debbie and Mike met with me together, as well. I gave them literature on more comfortable positions during intercourse, but, as the social worker had dealt with some of these issues, my role was limited. I did, however, discuss my concerns about Debbie's difficulties with heavy household tasks. Mike, who hadn't really thought much about this before these sessions, readily agreed to take on responsibility for these.

Debbie learned about a number of community resources. The local YMCA has activities tailored to people with arthritis. Our arthritis society sponsors a local support group that meets monthly to explore issues of common concern, and conducts a programme in arthritis self-management. It also has a telephone line that provides answers to questions about drugs, research and sources of equipment, and it produces a quarterly publication called *Arthritis News*. In the UK the principal charity is Arthritis Care (contact details in the 'Further resources' appendix), which has a network of over 500 branches or groups and an informative bi-monthly magazine, also called *Arthritis News*.

Surgery

Surgery plays an extremely important role in the treatment of people with arthritis. However, a surgical consultation is an admission of defeat. Something has happened, with me looking on, that I could not prevent.

These days, however, an admission of defeat doesn't mean a miserable future for the patient. Surgery has made enormous strides in the past 25 years.

When surgical help is sought, it's usually for one of three reasons:

- for relief of severe pain;

- for improved function;

- to try to prevent something from happening.

The first two objectives are most likely to be realised by surgery. Preventive surgery is carried out, however, in certain limited circumstances.

Broadly speaking, arthritis surgery divides into four types – joint replacement, joint fusion, reconstruction and soft tissue surgery.

Joint replacement

Joint replacement, pioneered in Britain in the late 1960s, has revolutionised orthopaedics, and bone and joint surgery. It's undoubtedly the greatest single contribution to the welfare of arthritis patients that has been made over the last three decades.

The first problem to be solved was OA of the hip. Although before the 1960s, artificial joints had been developed, there was no way to keep the parts from slipping. A new 'glue' solved the problem. Methyl methacrylate, a bone cement, proved to be a quick-setting, solid attachment for the metal parts, and the boom in joint replacement began.

Since then, the original techniques have been modified many times, because even with the discovery of bone cement there are still problems. The bond between bone and glue and metal does fail occasionally. The metal components themselves may ultimately fracture. If either happens, pain returns and eventually that joint has to be replaced. And second operations are never as good as first ones.

So new and stronger metal alloys have been developed. Special surface coatings have been bonded to metal to minimise body tissue reaction to these foreign substances. Components have been fabricated of new, porous materials, designed to encourage new bone to grow into the implanted parts, avoiding the use of glue and, it is hoped, providing an even stronger bond.

Total hip replacement (THR)

This operation was the first, and is still the best. Patients begin to put weight on the joint almost immediately after surgery, and the long-term results are excellent. At least 90 per cent of THRs are functioning well after 15 years. With today's models, 30 years of use is not an unreasonable expectation, unless the owner is grossly overweight or unusually physically active.

Total knee replacement (TKR)

This is almost as good as THR in terms of long-term outcome, although my impression is that a second operation, if necessary, is not as frequently or as completely successful as second THR surgery.

The only other major joints commonly replaced are shoulders and elbows.

Shoulder replacement

This is usually very successful for pain relief. As long as the ligaments and tendons around the shoulder (the 'rotator cuff') have not been severely damaged by the disease process, functional recovery is also quite good. Unfortunately, in RA the rotator cuff is frequently damaged and so pain relief, but usually not completely restored function, is the major goal of surgery.

Elbow replacement

This is done less frequently, and still has a long way to go. Movements of the elbow joint are complex. Unlike the hip and shoulder, the elbow is not protected by a thick covering of muscle. The older, 'hinge' type of elbow replacement was not very satisfactory and I only recommended it for patients with disabling pain. It didn't move like a real elbow, especially in twisting movements. But recently a three-piece elbow joint, looking very much like the three bones that come together at the elbow, has been developed. I've had a few patients who were delighted with the results – not just with the absence of pain but also with the improvement in function. I hope they continue to be just as happy as time and use test the limits of the hardware.

Deciding on surgery

When should joint replacement surgery be considered? That's a question that only the patient can answer. It really boils down to 'when pain or impaired function is at the point where daily life is becoming very difficult'. For two people with similar X-rays, that point might be quite different.

Surgery can be put off too long – particularly if the process has led to major bone loss or significant joint contracture (where the muscles and tendons around the joint became scarred and tight), or if a lot of muscle has been lost through lack of use. If an individual is off his or her feet for three months or more because of knee or hip arthritis, joint replacement surgery usually fails to correct the problem.

An orthopaedic consultation should take place before the patient reaches the point where surgery is urgent. That gives the patient and the surgeon a chance to size each other up. It allows time for a clear explanation of the risks and benefits, and for reflection. It also clears the way for a speedy surgical booking when, later, both patient and surgeon agree that the time has come.

Complications of joint replacement surgery

Complications are few. Infection is always a risk but the figure is now 1 per cent or less. If it occurs, the usual response is to operate again, take out the foreign material, clear the infection with antibiotics and start all over again. It's also recommended that, if patients later undergo procedures that may 'shower' bacteria into the bloodstream (and thence into the artificial joint), they be given a brief course of antibiotics. Dental surgery and passage of medical instruments into the bladder (cystoscopy) or colon (colonoscopy) are procedures of this type.

Phlebitis (inflammation with obstructing blood clots in the veins of the leg) is a major complication of hip, and to a lesser extent knee, replacement surgery. Because these clots can break loose, pass through the blood vessels to the lungs (pulmonary embolism) and even lead to death, this complication has been the subject of much research. Pulmonary embolism still occurs after approximately 2 per cent of hip operations, but the use of blood 'thinning' medication, at the time of surgery and after, has made a big difference.

Joint fusion

The goal of joint fusion, where a bony bridge is surgically constructed across a joint, is to relieve pain and to partially restore function where joint replacement is not possible.

This is most commonly carried out in the wrist and in the ankle region, and is most often done because of severe damage from RA. Total joint replacement surgery is not yet sufficiently developed to be used here. Fortunately, post-operative function is surprisingly reasonable, and the relief from pain here makes a huge difference.

Joints are also fused in two uncommon situations:

- Where total joint replacement has failed and repeat surgery is technically impossible.

- Where an artificial joint has been removed because of infection and repeat surgery would be extremely difficult or impossible.

Occasionally, the fusion of a single small joint (the middle joint of the thumb is a good example), converts a useless, unstable thumb into one that can function again in pinching and gripping.

Joint reconstruction

Technically speaking, total joint replacement fits into this category of surgery. However, what is referred to here is the surgical 'cleaning up' (debridement) of damaged bone ends, ligaments and tendons, followed by an attempt to reconstruct a functioning joint with the remaining tissues.

As might be guessed, the success rate of this effort varies. It depends on the disease that caused the damage, how much damage was done and how much work the reconstructed joint has to do.

In RA, this type of surgery is commonly done in the forefoot. The joints at the base of the toes, the MTP joints, are the target of prolonged inflammatory damage. As a result, the toes tend to slip upward into a 'hammer toe' position, taking with them the protective fat pad over the MTP joint and leaving the person to walk painfully on the damaged and inflamed bone ends. Reconstructive surgery involves removing the damaged metatarsal bone ends and the inflamed joint lining (the synovium), pulling the toes back down into alignment and tightening up the ligaments surrounding each joint. Problems with this type of surgery are twofold – a long healing period is necessary before full weight can be put on the foot, and the damage tends to gradually recur under the impact of continuing inflammation and the constant pounding the foot takes with every step.

Reconstructive surgery in the rheumatoid hand is more successful, at least from an appearance perspective. Such deformities as 'ulnar drift' of the fingers, and 'swan-neck' and 'boutonnière' knuckles, can be corrected. Whether the use of the hand is improved varies. Prior damage to the joints themselves, and to the small muscles that work the fingers, may be so extensive that the hand looks better but still doesn't work well.

Soft-tissue surgery

Soft-tissue surgery includes a variety of procedures. These are particularly common in RA, where local tissue inflammation can lead to a number of problems:

- In the shoulder, repair of rotator cuff tears (which cause shoulder weakness and pain).

- On the back of the wrist, removal of the thickened, heaped-up, inflamed tendon and joint lining (synovium) when it causes pain and when it threatens to lead to rupture of the tendons that straighten the fingers.

- On the inside of the wrist, when pressure on the median nerve causes numbness and tingling in the thumb and first three fingers ('carpal tunnel syndrome'), cutting of the tight ligament that pins the nerve down.

- Repair of finger tendons that have ruptured, and freeing of tendons that lock or seize up ('trigger fingers'), if local cortisone injections fail.

At one time, surgical removal of inflamed rheumatoid tissue from large joints such as the knee was felt to be both effective and necessary. This procedure, called a synovectomy, has been almost entirely abandoned. At best, it bought two years or more of freedom from inflammation in about 50 per cent of the joints, but at the cost of a major surgical procedure (including the risk of infection and phlebitis). There are perhaps two other reasons why it's fallen out of favour: general management of RA is much more effective, and results similar to surgical synovectomy can be achieved with the injection of a radioisotope into the knee.

Closed synovectomy through an arthroscope – a procedure that involves minimal damage to the muscles and ligaments that cover the joint – is a different matter. It is particularly useful if only one joint is inflamed, and if medicine by mouth or by injection into the joint has failed. A good example is the rare patient with Lyme disease who has persisting pain and swelling in a knee.

Treatment in pregnancy and breast-feeding

Many of my patients get pregnant, have babies and breast-feed. It would be unusual if this were not so, because many forms of arthritis, especially rheumatoid arthritis and systemic lupus erythematosus, target women in their childbearing years. These patients have three major concerns:

- What will be the effect of my pregnancy on my arthritis?
- What will be the effect of my arthritis on my pregnancy?
- Will drugs affect my baby?

The effect of pregnancy on arthritis

In RA the effect is usually favourable. At least half the women start to feel better within the first three months, and almost three-quarters experience marked improvement some time during the pregnancy. But a small minority will get worse – about 5 per cent – and the remainder will notice no change.

Unfortunately, after the baby is born, the inflammation returns. In nearly three out of four women this happens within the first two months. Most will have flared up by the end of six months, regardless of whether or not they are breast-feeding. It's distinctly unusual for RA to start during pregnancy, whereas it's not at all uncommon for it to begin following the birth of a child. It's almost as if pregnancy 'postpones' the disease, and it probably does.

It was the search for the cause of the benefits of pregnancy on RA that led Philip Hench to discover cortisone's effects. Although cortisone clearly has a powerful anti-inflammatory effect, Hench was wrong in believing that it was the reason pregnancy improved RA. The answer is much more complex, and is undoubtedly linked to the development of immune tolerance in the mother. This tolerance modifies her immune system to permit the baby, which is in effect a foreign tissue graft much like a transplanted kidney, to survive. In the process, the immune mechanisms that are responsible for so much in RA are suppressed.

Other forms of arthritis don't show such a clear-cut improvement with pregnancy. The few studies that have been done in psoriatic arthritis and ankylosing spondylitis suggest little or no benefit; some women improve, some stay the same and some worsen – in roughly equal numbers.

Pregnancy in systemic lupus erythematosus (SLE) has been studied extensively, but there does not appear to be any significant effect, for good or ill. Flare-ups of SLE do occur in pregnancy, but they occur at the same rate in similar patients who aren't pregnant. There aren't increased numbers of disease flare-ups or first appearances after delivery – unlike RA.

Carpal tunnel syndrome is common in pregnancy. Fluid retention and tissue swelling may matter little in most areas but in the carpal tunnel at the wrist they make a big difference. Pressure on the median nerve results in wrist and hand pain, numbness and tingling. Because body fluid tends to shift to the arms and hands at night, this is when the symptoms occur. The victim is awakened, and typically gets relief by hanging her arm over the side of the bed and shaking her hand vigorously. Relief comes with the birth of the baby, though a carpal tunnel splint worn on the wrist at night can help before then.

The effect of arthritis on pregnancy

Several studies have found an increased risk of miscarriages (spontaneous abortions) in mothers with RA. The expected rate of 10–15 per cent rises to about 25 per cent.

Active SLE carries with it a similar increased risk that the pregnancy will be lost. This risk can be reduced somewhat by avoiding pregnancy until the SLE is under good control. But in SLE there are additional factors that may affect pregnancy outcome.

Miscarriages occur not only in the 'usual' first trimester (up to 12 weeks) but also in the second trimester. Second-trimester loss is normally quite unusual, and in SLE it seems to be linked to the presence in the blood of the recently discovered 'anti-phospholipid antibody'. This factor is found in some people with SLE, as well as in otherwise healthy individuals. In both groups it's tied to delayed miscarriage. It's also linked to an increased risk of blood clot formation in veins (phlebitis) and, occasionally, arteries. There is still debate over what treatment best minimises the risk to both mother and baby if this blood factor is detected.

An additional and distinctly uncommon effect of SLE is on the developing infant heart. A different blood factor, 'anti-Ro antibody', has been linked to complete heart block (but not to an increased miscarriage rate). In this situation, the normal pathways that conduct the heart impulse are injured, causing a permanently slow heartbeat in the baby. This can be detected as early as the 16th week of pregnancy. Fortunately, normal heart action can be achieved nowadays by the implantation of an artificial pacemaker. This seems to be necessary in about half the affected babies.

Anti-Ro antibody also seems to play a role in the development of an SLE-like skin rash in some babies born to mothers carrying that factor. The factor, and the rash, disappears with the passage of time – at least by six months. It must be said, however, that most mothers with anti-Ro antibody will have normal babies.

Arthritis drugs and the baby, before and after birth

With good reason, most women avoid taking any type of medication during pregnancy. In some cases it's carried to the point where all drugs are stopped as soon as the woman decides to try to get pregnant. On the other hand, many women with arthritis who are taking a variety of drugs become pregnant unintentionally. From their experience, and from other situations, a number of conclusions can be reached.

- NSAIDs have not caused fetal abnormalities, and if they are essential they may be continued in early pregnancy.

- NSAIDs should be avoided in later pregnancy, particularly in the last few months. Aspirin, in particular, should be avoided because it has been linked to complications such as prolonged labour, bleeding after delivery and brain haemorrhage in the baby.

- NSAIDs can be taken during breast-feeding if needed. To minimise the baby's exposure, drugs with a short duration of action, such as ibuprofen, should be used. It has been calculated that, if the mother is taking ibuprofen, 400 milligrams four times a day, the baby receives less than 1 milligram. It has also been recommended that the medication be taken just as each breast-feeding session begins, assuming that the baby will not feed again for at least four hours.

- 'Slow-acting' drugs such as hydroxychloroquine, sulfasalazine, intramuscular gold and even azathioprine have not affected pregnancy adversely, even though there are theoretical ways they could harm the baby. The situation has to be weighed up very carefully, but if the drug is necessary to prevent a flare-up (particularly of SLE) it should be continued. A reduced dose might be tried as one way of cutting the risk. Both sulfasalazine and hydroxychloroquine have been used throughout pregnancy in non-arthritic situations, and seem to have a good record of safety.

- Prednisone may be the safest drug of all, particularly if only low doses are required.

- Cyclophosphamide and methotrexate are capable of great harm to the fetus and should never knowingly be taken during pregnancy, although normal pregnancies do occur even with these drugs.

Alternatives to conventional medicine

Not too long ago, nobody – neither I nor my patients – talked about this. Now just about all the patients I see ask me about something they've heard about from a neighbour, on television or on the internet. If I ask, they don't hesitate to tell me what they've tried, or are trying.

I wasn't surprised to read recently that in 1997 it was estimated that $27 billion was spent on 'alternative' medicine in the USA (Canada, at one-tenth the population, spends an estimated $3.8 billion Canadian). In one American city, two-thirds of people with appointments to see an arthritis specialist had tried at least one 'unconventional' treatment, a quarter had tried three or more and at least half who had tried one were continuing to use it.

The variety of treatments is astounding – chiropractic, copper bracelets, magnets, herbs, electrical stimulators, diet supplements and special diets, minerals and megavitamins, vinegar preparations, acupuncture and spiritual healing. Despite the variety, most of these treatments have one thing in common – they haven't been proved scientifically to help the problem for which the person is using them.

A wise doctor once said, 'There is no such thing as alternative medicine – just effective medicine.'

It seems clear that many patients choose to pursue two paths at the same time – the 'conventional' path I recommend, and the 'alternative' path, usually on the grounds that it can't hurt and may help. Use of alternative treatments may also be a marker for significant psychological distress, often depression; this is true of some women with breast cancer, and it may be true for people with arthritis as well.

I want to make it clear that I don't criticise a patient who wishes to pursue one of these approaches. I've been around medicine long enough to realise that allopathic medicine (the kind of medicine I practice) has no monopoly on truth – or on untruth.

Dr Michael Lockshin, a New York rheumatologist and former chair of the Unproven Remedies Committee of the Arthritis Foundation, says people should ask themselves three questions about unproven treatments:

- 'Will it hurt me?'

- 'Will it cost me a lot of money?'

- 'Will it help?'

If I can be sure the answer to the first two is no, I often encourage my patients to find out the answer to the third. I just hope they won't ignore a proven treatment at the same time.

Diet and arthritis

Should something be dropped from the diet?

Food allergies are widespread. An extremely conservative estimate is that about 2 per cent of the population have an unmistakable food allergy. Egg, wheat, milk, fish and shellfish, nuts, chocolate and citrus fruits are some of the common offenders. Allergic symptoms cover a wide spectrum, from hay fever and asthma symptoms to skin rash, including hives, to gut upset and migraine, to muscle and joint aches and pains, and even, in extreme cases, death.

There have been clear-cut instances where arthritis symptoms in people diagnosed as having RA have come and gone in response to the addition and withdrawal of specific foods given in a 'double-blind' fashion. The foods varied by patient, and included corn, wheat, nitrate, shrimp and milk. Most of these people seemed to be rheumatoid factor (RF) negative. But estimates of the number of RA patients whose symptoms are affected by food are well under 5 per cent.

In isolated instances, flare-ups of childhood arthritis and SLE have been linked to specific foods.

A different kind of example is coeliac disease, a condition where people are intolerant of gluten, a protein found in wheat, rye, barley and, to some extent, oats. Coeliacs often have musculoskeletal symptoms – some quite severe – which improve on a gluten-free diet. I well recall a young woman with intractable pain who, after several years of fruitless investigations and treatment at my hands, saw another doctor who made the correct diagnosis and cured her with changes to her diet.

A number of special diets have been studied. Most of these, done in patients with RA, started with a period of fasting (often up to a week); then various foods were reintroduced, with or without attempts to avoid specific items. In some instances, a tailored kind of diet was started. The results of these studies have been mixed. Some have shown no benefit. Many others have shown definite benefit, especially during the fasting phase.

One of the most convincing of these demonstrated that a small minority of patients were clearly helped by a diet that eliminated red meat, dairy products, alcohol, preservatives, fruit, herbs and spices. A slightly different study found that 17 patients put on a long-term vegetarian diet improved and were able to maintain their improvement for at least a year. But nutritionists examining this study have criticised it for two reasons: the numbers were very small, and the diet itself had nutritional deficiencies that could lead to difficulty in the long run.

The conclusion to draw from all of this? There is no blanket prescription. A small number of individuals – probably very few – have food allergies that cause symptoms. In other instances, a vegetarian-type diet may modestly improve the signs and symptoms of inflammation. But medical research continues in this area. I don't think we've heard the last word on dietary manipulation.

Should something be added to the diet?
Zinc, selenium, copper and vitamins B and C have all been investigated. Addition of these does not affect arthritis.

Eicosapentaenoic acid (EPA) and gammalinolenic acid (GLA) have been shown experimentally to be anti-inflammatory and to blunt immune responses. Fish oils, including cod liver oil, contain EPA. Plant oils, specifically oils from evening primrose and borage, contain GLA. Theoretically, blackcurrant seed oil is even better, because it contains both GLA and a chemical that is converted to EPA.

Studies with these oils have found that they definitely reduce the 'tenderness and pain' index in RA, and may affect the extent of the swelling as well. But studies so far have looked only at high doses. It remains to be seen whether lower doses, which would be much easier to take, will be as good.

The extract of the New Zealand green-lipped mussel (Seatone) seems to have some anti-inflammatory effect in the test-tube and in rats. But well-designed studies haven't turned up any evidence of effectiveness in people with rheumatoid or osteoarthritis. And it's expensive.

In the last few years, three dietary supplements – glucosamine (with or without chondroitin), SAMe and MSM – have become popular. I have already commented on glucosamine – it clearly helps many with the pain of osteoarthritis, but has never been shown to be effective in inflammatory arthritis. SAMe ('sammy' or S-adenosyl methionine) is an antidepressant and early studies support claims for it as a pain reliever. It has also been recommended as an anti-arthritic – but without proof, at least so far. At the recommended dosage 4 to 16 caplets a day, it is expensive. Finally, MSM, which is a breakdown product of dimethyl sulfoxide (DMSO), is being promoted in Canada by a great deal of advertising and word-of-mouth enthusiasm as an arthritis cure. I haven't seen any convincing studies, however, and until I do I'm not going to be recommending it to anyone – certainly not if I think there is a more effective, proven treatment available.

Herbal remedies

'All who drink of this remedy are cured, except those who die. Thus it is effective for all but the incurable.'

GALEN (AD 130–201)

Despite their immense popularity – herbs are, of course, 'natural' products and therefore often assumed to be 'quite safe' – herbal remedies have not been proved effective in arthritis.

There are many good reasons not to take herbal remedies. Poisoning is one, and it isn't rare. Some cases arise because of contamination and misidentification, but most are probably related to the natural chemistry of the plants themselves. Infants and children seem to be particularly vulnerable.

Another strong reason to be careful with herbal remedies is their potential to interact with conventional drugs for such problems as heart failure, irregular heartbeat patterns, high blood pressure, blood clots, seizures and depression. As a result, conventional drugs may lose their effect – or may have a stronger effect, resulting in a drug overdose.

Some herbal remedies that may be particularly worrisome are gingko, ginseng, feverfew, St John's wort, ma-huang (Chinese ephedra), devil's claw and plantain. Echinacea, recommended as an immune system stimulant, may be just what someone on immunosuppressive treatment for RA or SLE doesn't need.

Don't forget that herbs are drugs. Until the active ingredients of a herbal preparation are known, and it is established that the preparation contains a known concentration of them, be careful – especially if you are taking conventional drugs. Check with a pharmacist – most should have good information on potential harmful interactions.

In most Western countries, including Canada, the USA and the UK, herbal remedies are classified as foods and don't have to pass the more stringent regulations applied to drugs.

Quality control seems to be a big problem. Analysis has found some preparations to be adulterated with other drugs, and with heavy metals. This is particularly true of products for which there's a huge market – and many unscrupulous individuals wishing to share it.

'Chinese herbal medicines' may contain a variety of herbs and contaminating substances. Deaths due to liver failure, sudden drop in blood pressure and kidney failure have been reported.

Chinese proprietary medicines deserve special mention. These are very popular, not only in the Far East. An elderly Chinese lady with RA is a patient of mine. She has taken Chinese proprietary medicines for some time – she gets them from relatives in Hong Kong. She's delighted with their effect, and won't hear of stopping them. I did persuade her to bring me the package, and printed on the side were the ingredients of each tablet – a cortisone-like drug, two different NSAIDs (one restricted in Canada) and a pain-killer. Some of these ingredients were in laughably low doses, others in doses higher than I would use. Similar preparations obtainable in Hong Kong and presumably contaminated (I hope hers isn't) have been linked to mercury, lead, cadmium and arsenic poisoning.

Periodically, I discover that a patient has obtained some arthritis remedy from Mexico. When these have been analysed, they too have invariably contained cortisone-like drugs and an NSAID – a combination with high risk for side effects.

Finally, let me say something positive about herbal remedies. Many have been around a very long time. Tradition does say something about safety and effectiveness. We just need to know more about them. We need to isolate the chemicals unique to each herb and test them carefully, first in the laboratory and then in the clinic.

A good example of this is the Chinese herb known as thunder god vine, a remedy that has been used for years in China to treat RA. Its active ingredient – triptolide – has been isolated. It has now been tested in the lab and found to keep immune cells from turning on the inflammation chain reaction (it may also have anti-cancer actions). The leap from the lab to the pharmacy is a big one but, if tests in humans prove successful, we may soon have another weapon to use against such conditions as RA and SLE.

Acupuncture

In 1972 – coincident with Richard Nixon's trip to China – the Western world 'discovered' acupuncture. The theory of acupuncture attributes illness to an imbalance of body energy forces. Based on an assessment of this imbalance, needles are inserted beneath the skin according to a predetermined pattern. The pattern is dictated by which 'meridian' of the body system was out of balance, as well as by the influences – Wind, Cold, Fire, Dampness, Dryness and Summer Heat – that might be affecting this imbalance.

I think I can safely make several statements about acupuncture:

- It has never been shown to cure any disease.

- When needle placement is made at traditional Chinese locations, a pain-relieving effect can be detected.

- This pain-relieving effect is superior to the effect (which can also be detected) of needle placement in nearby sites which are not those prescribed by traditional Chinese practice.

- Acupuncture needle stimulation in experimental animals causes release of natural pain-killers (endorphins).

- Acupuncture seems to have a definite role in the treatment of both acute and chronic musculoskeletal pain. Studies of long-standing low back pain have been particularly impressive.

- It seems to work best when it's co-ordinated with a variety of other approaches – physiotherapy, fitness and muscle strengthening, lifestyle changes.

* There are various schools of acupuncture. None has shown its superiority over any other.

My advice? Acupuncture is worth a try, particularly if you're attempting to deal with long-standing, disabling, non-inflammatory pain. Just don't give up on the other things I also recommend, and go only to fully trained acupuncturists.

Homoeopathy

Homoeopathy is based on the 'Law of Similars'. The first principle of homoeopathy holds that a condition can be treated by administering a substance which, in full strength, causes symptoms similar to the disease to be treated. An 18th-century German physician, Samuel Hahnemann, popularised this principle after taking a strong dose of cinchona bark – which contains the antimalarial quinine – and experiencing headache, thirst and fever – all symptoms of malaria. With friends, he began experimenting with various herbs and other substances, making careful notes on the symptoms produced. He then moved on to develop the second principle of homoeopathy – that if a large dose of a substance causes symptoms of a given disease, then extremely small doses will cure it. The smaller the dose, the stronger the medicine.

The difficulty most conventional doctors have with the theory is that the dilutions are carried to such an extreme that the laws of chemistry make it infinitely unlikely that any given bottle will contain a single molecule of the substance. A standard '30C' strength of saline, for instance, is comparable to one molecule of salt dissolved in a volume of water equivalent to all this planet's waters. But homoeopathy rises above the mathematics. It concludes that the alcohol or water of the solution develops a 'memory' of the substance to which it has been exposed, and that it's this 'memory' that has the desired effect.

So much for the theory. Does homoeopathy work? Again we come to controlled studies, and again the data just aren't there. There has been only one acceptable study in RA. In contrast to a number of other reports that showed no benefit, it demonstrated a reduction in pain in patients receiving homoeopathic treatment. This study has been criticised on the grounds that the patients weren't assigned in a random fashion to one group or the other, and so it does not meet strict study criteria.

To be fair, there have been a very few studies that were well designed and showed treatment benefits in flu, hay fever and infant diarrhoea. But, like any research results, these should be repeated successfully before they are fully accepted.

In the meantime, while I certainly wouldn't recommend them, homoeopathic remedies seem harmless enough – as long as using them doesn't mean postponing treatment that is known to be effective.

Chiropractic

The most common symptom for which people seek alternative medicine is back pain. And the most commonly sought out alternative practitioner is the chiropractor.

In 1990 the *British Medical Journal* reported on two groups of patients with low back pain. One group was treated by chiropractors, one by physiotherapists. At the end of two years, the chiropractic-treated group felt better – but they had been treated more intensively, at a greater cost, over the two years. Nevertheless, this outcome was viewed as a vindication of those who advocated chiropractic.

More recently, the *New England Journal of Medicine* reported a two-year study of similar low-back-pain sufferers. Here, though, there were three groups – a chiropractic group, a physiotherapy group and a group that was given an educational pamphlet on low back pain. The outcome was similar in all three groups – particularly in terms of days off work, reduced activity and return of pain. The booklet group had slightly but not significantly more symptoms, but was definitely less happy (30 per cent happy) about the treatment given, compared to the other two groups (75 per cent happy).

What do I conclude from all this? Back pain gets better in almost anyone, but the laying on of hands – by a chiropractor or a physiotherapist – makes people happier. That is no mean achievement, and I don't hesitate to recommend one or the other to my patients. But first I make sure that the back pain is not a signal of an underlying condition in which delay or chiropractic manipulation would be harmful.

And all the rest

Regular newspaper readers will recognise WD-40 oil, DMSO (dimethyl sulfoxide), copper bracelets, bee venom, honey and vinegar, and sitting in abandoned radium mines as all making claims to effectiveness in arthritis. Unfortunately, at this time that's all they are. Claims.

I don't pretend to have all the answers. I recognise that the theory behind a lot of what we have done in arthritis treatment has been faulty, and that quite a lot of what was done not so very long ago was worthless and even harmful.

The best I can do is attempt to evaluate current practice honestly, tell my patients what we do and don't know, and let them decide. If they decide to pursue unconventional medicine, as long as they do it with full knowledge of the uncertainties and the alternatives, I can't criticise their choice.

'I didn't say there was nothing better,' the King replied.
'I said there was nothing like it.'

LEWIS CARROLL, *Through the Looking Glass.*

Glossary

Some definitions refer to 'skeleton' – see the diagram preceding Chapter 1.

acute In a medical context, short term (see also *chronic*)

anaemia A condition in which the number of red blood cells (responsible for carrying oxygen from the lungs to body tissues) is lower than normal. The two most common reasons for anaemia are (1) excessive blood loss (such as from a bleeding stomach ulcer) and (2) defective manufacture of new blood cells (which is a common problem in many chronic diseases). Both may contribute to anaemia in some forms of arthritis.

antibody A protein molecule, made by a specialised white blood cell (the B-lymphocyte). Antibodies are normally custom-made to help protect the body against foreign proteins (known as antigens). The body encounters many antigens every day – viruses, bacteria, drugs are some. In some forms of arthritis, antibodies are formed against normal body proteins and disease symptoms may result from this 'autoimmune' reaction. Rheumatoid factor (RF) is an auto-antibody of this type.

arthralgia Pain in one or many joints (used when swelling is not observed).

arthroplasty Surgery carried out on a joint in an attempt to improve its function. Artificial joint surgery, such as a total knee arthroplasty, fits into this category.

arthroscopy A procedure that involves introducing a small-diameter flexible fibreoptic cable, through the skin, into a joint. This allows the interior of the joint to be examined. Almost any joint can be examined in this fashion, but the knee is the most common. Surgery can also be performed at the same time by introducing similarly small instruments into the joint and operating under 'direct arthroscopic vision'.

bursa A sac-like structure found over many places on the body where pressure is applied. Many bursae are just beneath the skin (such as the olecranon bursa, covering the tip of the elbow) and others are deeper. A bursa in its normal 'collapsed' state is similar to a small deflated balloon that contains a few drops of fluid. It allows the overlying tissues to roll over the bony bump without tearing. If the bursa is injured or inflamed, it may swell and become tense and painful – a condition called bursitis.

cartilage The tough whitish covering of the ends of bones where they come together in a joint. Cartilage permits smooth, low-friction movement. When it deteriorates, the process known as osteoarthritis develops.

chronic Long-term or long-lasting (see also *acute*)

claudication Leg pain coming on when the blood supply can't provide the necessary oxygen to the exercising muscles. It is relieved by resting the muscles or by doing something (usually surgical) to improve the circulation. One form of back disease (spinal stenosis) can cause pain very similar to vascular claudication.

collagen The most abundant protein in the body, usually formed in thick tough strands, that provides strength and shape to many body structures, including cartilage, skin and heart valve tissues.

connective tissue disease A term that is about as meaningless as 'arthritis'. Connective tissue consists of the cells, fibres (including collagen) and semi-liquid 'glue' that hold tissues together. At one point about 30 years ago, it was proposed that the common denominator in a wide variety of conditions (including rheumatoid arthritis, systemic lupus erythematosus, polymyositis and scleroderma) was a defect in connective tissue. It's still used as a useful shorthand for referring to such diseases but shouldn't be taken to imply that connective tissue is anything more than an innocent bystander.

COX An enzyme, cyclo-oxygenase, that initiates the production of inflammatory chemicals. COX is the target for the NSAID group of drugs.

CT (or CAT) scan The acronym stands for 'computed axial tomography'. This is a process whereby the technology of X-ray and that of the computer are combined, producing an image of body tissues previously unavailable. We use it in rheumatology to look at bone and, in particular, the spine.

dactylitis Dactyls are fingers and toes. Inflammation may cause individual toes or fingers to become diffusely swollen and red – hence 'dactylitis'.

DIP joints The joints at the ends of the fingers. DIP = distal interphalangeal (see skeleton).

disc (or disk) The 'cushion' between individual vertebrae, or bones of the spine. Its outer layers consist of thick strands of tightly wound collagen, like the outer layers of a golf ball, and – like a golf ball – its centre is a semi-liquid gel. This permits the disc to act as a 'shock-absorber'. With age, the centre of the disc tends to dry up, causing a shrinkage in disc height.

enthesis The point where ligaments and tendons attach to bone. Inflammation at this point is called an 'enthesitis'. A 'tennis elbow' and a 'heel spur' are examples of enthesitis.

epicondyles The bony 'knobs' on the inside and the outside of the elbow joint (where the forearm muscles are attached).

fascia A tough sheet of tissue, usually just under the skin, which covers and protects underlying structures. One such layer covers the outside of the thigh from pelvis to knee; another covers the sole of the foot from the base of the toes to the heel. 'Fasciitis' refers to inflammation of this tissue.

intra-articular Literally, within the joint.

isometric exercise Exercising by contracting the muscles without significant joint movement, usually done against resistance.

lumbar/lumbosacral Refers to the lower five vertebrae of the spine (the lumbar spine). Lumbosacral extends the reference to include the sacrum, the curved segment at the base of the spine (see skeleton).

MCP joints The joints at the base of the fingers that form the near row of knuckles. MCP = metacarpophalangeal (see skeleton).

microsurgery Surgery carried out with the help of a magnifying apparatus. In bone and joint surgery, microsurgical disc surgery is sometimes carried out in an attempt to be less injurious to the surrounding tissues.

monarticular Literally, involving a single joint.

MTP joints The joints at the base of the toes that form the 'ball' of the foot. MTP = metatarsophalangeal (see skeleton).

musculoskeletal Refers to muscles, bones and joints.

NSAID An acronym for non-steroidal anti-inflammatory drug(s), pronounced 'ensaid'. It includes aspirin and a host of others such as ibuprofen, indometacin and naproxen. Pain-killers such as paracetamol are not NSAIDs.

OA The acronym for 'osteoarthritis'.

occupational therapy One of the health professions involved in helping people with arthritis adapt to their disease and their environment (see Chapter 7).

oedema The accumulation of increased, and abnormal, amounts of water in body tissues. The swelling of ankles and feet during pregnancy is due to oedema.

orthopaedic An adjective that refers to the correct positioning of the skeleton. Orthopaedic surgery is the branch of surgery that aims at correcting skeletal disorders, including fractures and the damage done by arthritis.

orthotic A device, such as a splint or insole, designed to support a part of the skeleton in its normal position or posture.

osteoporosis A condition in which the solidity of bone is greatly reduced by an excess of normal bone breakdown over bone repair (see the section 'Cortisone' in Chapter 7).

osteotomy A surgical incision into bone, designed to change its alignment.

phlebitis Inflammation of a vein. When this is accompanied by the development of a blood clot (thrombosis) in the inflamed segment of vein, as it often is, the term 'thrombophlebitis' is used.

physiotherapy A method of treatment designed to restore function in the musculoskeletal system. Strong emphasis is placed on exercise.

PIP joints Proximal interphalangeal (PIP) joints form the 'middle' knuckles halfway down the fingers and toes.

plantar Refers to the bottom of the foot. In the hand, the equivalent term is 'palmar'.

polyarthritis Literally, 'many (poly-) joints (arthr-) inflamed (itis)'. This is usually qualified by an adjective such as 'seronegative' (i.e. the rheumatoid factor test is negative) or 'symmetrical' (that is, both sides of the body are similarly affected).

prosthesis A replacement for a normal body part (in orthopaedic surgery, this may mean anything from an artificial joint to an artificial leg).

RA The acronym for 'rheumatoid arthritis'.

rheumatoid factor An antibody found in the blood in about 5 per cent of the normal population, but found in the blood of 60 per cent or more of people who have rheumatoid arthritis (and sometimes other forms of arthritis as well).

rheumatologist A medical doctor who specialises in the prevention, diagnosis and non-surgical treatment of the many forms of arthritis.

seropositive Medical jargon that implies that the blood test for a condition was positive (a patient can be 'seropositive' for HIV, or mononucleosis, or syphilis – but in people with arthritis it usually is taken to mean that the blood test for rheumatoid factor is positive).

SLE The acronym for 'systemic lupus erythematosus'.

spondylarthritis The variety of inflammatory arthritis that affects the spine and, often, the joints of the arms and legs. Ankylosing spondylitis and psoriatic arthritis are examples.

synovium The membrane lining the joint. It makes the lubricating fluid of the joint, and in inflammatory arthritis it becomes very inflamed and thickened and plays an important role in the joint damage that occurs.

systemic Refers to conditions in which more than one – usually many – of the body's organ systems are affected.

tophus (plural: **tophi**) A mass of crystals of sodium urate, collected together in a 'lump' under the skin, that may be detected in individuals with gout.

Further resources

Books

Aladjem, Henrietta. *The Challenges of Lupus: Insights and Hope.* New York, NY: Avery, 1999

Aladjem, Henrietta. *Understanding Lupus.* New York, NY: Scribner, 1985

Gach, Michael Reed. *Arthritis Relief at your Fingertips.* London: Piatkus, 1993

Hall, Hamilton. *The Back Doctor.* Toronto, ON: Seal, 1982

Hills, Margaret. *Curing Arthritis: More ways to a drug free life.* London: Sheldon Press, 1991

Holford, Patrick. *Say No to Arthritis* (Optimum Nutrition Handbook). London: Piatkus, 2000

Horstman, Judith. *The Arthritis Foundation's Guide to Alternative Therapies.* Marietta, GA: Longstreet Press, 1999

Hunder, Gene (ed.). *Mayo Clinic on Arthritis.* New York, NY: Kensington, 1999

Lorig, Kate, and James N. Fries. *The Arthritis Helpbook*, 4th edition. Reading, MA: Perseus, 1995

Nelson, Miriam E. *Strong Men and Women Beat Arthritis.* London: Aurum Press, 2003

Shlotzhauer, Tammi, and James McGuire (eds.). *Living with Rheumatoid Arthritis* (Johns Hopkins Health Book). Baltimore, MD: Johns Hopkins, 1995

Sobel, Dava, and Klein, Arthur C. *Arthritis.* London: Constable Robinson, 1998

de Vries, Jan. *Arthritis, Rheumatism and Psoriasis.* Edinburgh: Mainstream, 2002

Wallace, Daniel. *The Lupus Book: A Guide for Patients and Their Families.* New York, NY: Oxford, 1996

Wallace, Daniel, and Janice Wallace. *Making Sense of Fibromyalgia.* New York, NY: Oxford, 1999

Youngson, Robert. *Coping Successfully with Rheumatism and Arthritis.* London: Sheldon Press, 1998

Useful organisations and websites

Age Concern England
1268 London Road
London SW16 4ER
Tel: 020 8765 7200
Fax: 020 8765 7211
Website: www.ageconcern.org.uk
*Works on behalf of older people,
with advice and a range of
information leaflets and
publications, including caring
for someone with arthritis.*

Arthritis Care
18 Stephenson Way
London NW1 2HD
Helplines: 0800 800 4050
(Mon–Fri, noon–4pm)
020 7380 6555
(Mon–Fri, 10am–4pm)
Helpline for young people:
0808 808 2000
(Mon–Fri, 10am–2pm)
Fax: 020 7380 6505
Website: www.arthritiscare.org.uk
*Provides information and support
to enable people to live with and
manage arthritis. Campaigns for
greater awareness and better
services. The helpline is the first
port of call for anyone with
arthritis. Many small organisations
for particular types of arthritis;
for details ring the helpline or
Freephone 0808 800 4050*

Arthritis Foundation
of Ireland
1 Clanwilliam Square
Grand Canal Quay
Dublin 2
Ireland

Tel: 00 353 1 66 18188
Fax: 00 353 1 66 18261
Website: www.arthritis-foundation.com
*General information and support
with educational lectures. Local
support groups run information
and fundraising events.*

Arthritis Research
Campaign
Copeman House
St Mary's Court
St Mary's Gate
Chesterfield S41 7TD
Tel: 01246 558 033
Fax: 01246 558 007
Website: www.arc.org.uk
*Finances an extensive programme
of research and education in a
wide range of arthritis and
rheumatism problems, including
back pain. Has useful booklets
explaining related problems and
ways of coping with them.*

BackCare
16 Elmtree Road
Teddington TW11 8ST
Tel: 020 8977 5474
Fax: 020 8943 5318
Website: www.backcare.org.uk
*Information and advice for
people with back pain. Funds
patient-orientated scientific
research into the causes, treatment
and prevention of back pain.
Has local support groups
throughout the country with
regular meetings.*

Benefits Enquiry Line

Tel: 0800 88 22 00
Northern Ireland: 0800 220 674
Textphone: 0800 243 355
Website: www.dwp.gov.uk
*Government agency giving
information about state benefits
for sick or disabled people and
their carers.*

British Acupuncture Council

63 Jeddo Road
London W12 9HQ
Tel: 020 8735 0400
Fax: 020 8735 0404
Website: www.acupuncture.org.uk
*Professional body offering lists of
qualified acupuncture therapists.*

British Homeopathic Association

Hahnemann House
29 Park Street West
Luton LU1 3BE
Tel: 08704 443 950
Fax: 08704 443 960
Website: www.trusthomeopathy.org
*Professional body offering lists of
qualified homoeopathic
practitioners.*

British Society for Rheumatology

41 Eagle Street
London WC1R 4TL
Tel: 020 7242 3313
Fax: 020 7242 3277
Website: www.rheumatology.org.uk
*Professional membership body
representing rheumatologists.*

Carers UK

20–25 Glasshouse Yard
London EC1A 4JS
Helpline: 0808 808 7777
(Mon–Fri, 10am–noon; 2–4pm)
Tel: 020 7490 8818
Fax: 020 7490 8824
Website: www.carersonline.org.uk
*Provides a wide range of
information and support to all
carers.*

Chartered Society of Physiotherapy

14 Bedford Road
London WC1R 4ED
Tel: 020 7306 6666
Fax: 020 7306 6611
Website: www.csp.org.uk
*For information about all aspects
of physiotherapy; offers list of
chartered physiotherapists in your
area.*

Children's Chronic Arthritis Association

Ground Floor
Amber Gate
City Wall Road
Worcester WR1 2AH
Tel: 01905 745 595
Fax: 01905 745 703
Website: www.ccaa.org.uk
*Offers practical information to
maximise choices and
opportunities and raise awareness
of childhood arthritis in the
community. A support network
run by parents offers emotional
support; runs a yearly family
week-end conference.*

Department of Health
PO Box 777
London SE1 6HX
Helpline: 0800 555 777
Tel: 020 7210 4850
Textphone: 020 7210 3000
Fax: 01623 724 524
Website: www.doh.gov.uk
*Produces literature about all
health issues, including
prescription charges and
prepayment certificates, available
via the Helpline. A more technical
site, with National Service
Frameworks, is available at
www.doh.gov.uk/nsf/arthritis.*

Department for Work and Pensions
Benefits Enquiry Line:
0800 88 22 00
Tel: 020 7712 2171
Textphone: 0800 24 33 55
Fax: 020 7712 2386
Website: www.dwp.gov.uk
*Government department giving
information about, and claim
forms for, all state benefits.*

Disability Alliance
Universal House
88–94 Wentworth Street
London E1 7SA
Helpline: 020 7247 8765 (Mon &
Wed, 2–4pm)
Tel: 020 7247 8776 (voice and
textphone)
Fax: 020 7247 8763
Website: www.disabilityalliance.org
*Information on welfare benefits
entitlement, to people with
disabilities, their families, carers
and professional advisers.*

*Services include advice, campaign
work, research and training.*

Disability Sport England
N17 Studio, Unit 4G
784–788 High Road
London N17 0DA
Tel: 020 8801 4466
Fax: 020 8801 6644
Website: www.disabilitysport.org.uk
*National events agency that
encourages sport for people of all
ages with disabilities from local to
national level.*

Disabled Drivers Association
National Headquarters
Ashwellthorpe
Norwich NR16 1EX
Tel: 0870 770 3333
Fax: 01508 488 173
Website: www.dda.org.uk
*Self-help association offering
information and advice and
aiming for independence through
mobility.*

Disabled Living Centres Council
Redbank House
4 St Chad's Street
Manchester M8 8QA
Tel: 0161 834 1044
Textphone: 0161 839 0885
Fax: 0161 839 0802
Website: www.dlcc.org.uk
*For a Centre near you, where you
can see furniture, aids and equip-
ment for elderly and disabled
people. Offers training courses for
health professionals; information
leaflets available on request.*

Disabled Living Foundation

380–384 Harrow Road
London W9 2HU
Helpline: 0845 130 1977
Tel: 020 7289 6111
Textphone: 020 7432 8009
Fax: 020 7266 2922
Website: www.dlf.org.uk
Provides information to disabled and elderly people on all kinds of equipment in order to promote their independence and quality of life.

European League against Rheumatism (EULAR)

Eular Executive Secretariat
Witikonerstrasse 15
CH 8032 Zurich, Switzerland
Tel: + 41 1 383 9690
Fax: + 41 1 383 9810
Website: www.eular.org
Publishes journals, holds international conferences; website shows images of different diseases. Provides up-to-date information for professionals and patient organisations.

Fibromyalgia Association UK

PO Box 206
Stourbridge DY9 8YL
Tel: 0870 220 1232
Fax: 0870 752 5118
Website:
www.fibromyalgia-associationuk.org
Provides information for patients with fibromyalgia and has a network of local support groups throughout the UK. Campaigns for a better recognition and awareness of the disorder.

General Osteopathic Council

Osteopathy House
176 Tower Bridge Road
London SE1 3LU
Tel: 020 7357 6655
Fax: 020 7357 0011
Website: www.osteopathy.org.uk
Regulatory body that offers information to the public and lists of accredited osteopaths.

Help the Aged

207–221 Pentonville Road
London N1 9UZ
Tel: 020 7278 1114
Helpline: 0808 80 6565
Fax: 020 7278 1116
Website: www.helptheaged.org.uk
Offers advice and a range of free information leaflets on benefits, community and residential care and housing options.

Hypermobility Syndrome Association

PO Box 1122
Nailsea
Bristol BS48 2YZ
Website: www.hypermobility.org
Provides information and support via its members to others affected by this distressing 'hidden disorder'. Promotes knowledge and understanding within the medical community and the public at large through literature and videos. Holds yearly residential week-ends for members. Please send SAE for information.

Independent Living Fund

PO Box 7525
Nottingham NG2 4ZT
Helpline: 0845 601 8815
Tel: 0115 942 8191
Fax: 0115 945 0948
Website: www.ilf.org.uk
May provide top-up funding for very severely disabled people to buy in extra personal and/or domestic care. Applicants must already be receiving the higher care allowance and at least £200 care package from Social Services. Referral via Social Services.

International League of Associations for Rheumatology

Dr A O Adebajo
Academic Department of Rheumatology
Division of Genomic Medicine, M Floor
Royal Hallamshire Hospital
Beech Hill Road
Sheffield S10 2SB
Website: www.ilar.org
An umbrella body representing international organisations that hold conferences for health professionals.

Joint Zone

Website: www.jointzone.org.uk
Free educational website, funded by the Arthritis Research Campaign, International League of Associations for Rheumatology and others, intended mainly for medical students, with information about various forms of arthritis and treatments. Gives case studies and lectures.

MAVIS (Mobility Advice and Vehicle Information Service)

Department for Transport
Crowthorne Business Estate
Old Wokingham Road
Crowthorne
Berkshire RG45 6XD
Tel: 01344 661000
Fax: 01344 661066
Website: www.mobility-unit.dft.gov.uk
Government department offering driving and vehicle assessments and advice for people with mobility problems. Can advise on vehicle adaptations for both drivers and passengers.

Motability

Goodman House
Station Approach
Harlow
Essex CM20 2ET
Helpline: 01279 635 666
(8.45am–5.15pm, Mon–Fri)
Tel: 01279 635 999 (admin)
Textphone: 01279 632 273
Fax: 01279 632 000
Website: www.motability.co.uk
Advises people with disabilities about powered wheelchairs, scooters, and new and used cars, how to adapt them to their needs and how to obtain funding via the Mobility Scheme.

National Ankylosing Spondylitis Society (NASS)

PO Box 179
Mayfield
East Sussex TN20 6ZL
Tel: 01435 873 527
Fax: 01435 873 027
Web: www.nass.co.uk
Provides information and advice to patients with ankylosing spondylitis, their families and professionals. Has over 100 branches providing supervised physiotherapy one evening a week. Video and cassette tapes of physiotherapy exercises available.

National Centre for Independent Living

250 Kennington Lane
London SE11 5RD
Tel: 020 7587 1663
Textphone: 020 7587 1177
Fax: 020 7582 2469
Website: www.ncil.org.uk
Provides advice on independent living and Direct Payments, and details of your local Centre for Independent Living, to enable people to buy private personal and/or domestic care instead of receiving it via the local authority.

NHS Direct

Tel: 0845 46 47
Textphone: 0845 606 4647
NHS24 (Scotland): 0800 22 44 88
Website: www.nhsdirect.nhs.uk
First point of contact to find out about NHS services and for any health advice, which is available 24 hours daily, 365 days a year.

National Osteoporosis Society

Camerton
Bath
Somerset BA2 0PJ
Helpline: 0845 450 0230
Tel: 01761 471 771
Fax: 01761 471 104
Website: www.nos.org.uk
Provides information and advice on all aspects of osteoporosis, the menopause and hormone replacement therapy. Encourages people to take action to protect their bones. Helpline staffed by specially trained nurses. Has local support groups.

Pain Society

21 Portland Place
London W1B 1PY
Tel: 020 7631 8870
Fax: 020 7323 2015
Website: www.painsociety.org
Primarily for health care professionals; publishes Understanding and Managing Pain *for patients.*

Patients Association

PO Box 935
Harrow
Middlesex HA1 3YJ
Helpline: 0845 608 4455
(Mon–Fri, 10am–4pm)
Tel (admin): 020 8423 9111
(Mon–Fri, 9am–5pm)
Fax: 020 8423 9119
Website: www.patients-association.com
Gives advice on patients' rights, complaints procedures and access to health services or appropriate self-help groups.

Psoriatic Arthropathy Alliance

PO Box 111
St Albans AL2 3JQ
Tel: 0870 770 3212
Fax: 0870 770 3213
Website: www.paalliance.org
Raises awareness of psoriatic arthropathy. Provides informa-tion, produces a regular journal and puts people in touch with one another. You don't have to be a member if you wish to receive information.

RADAR (Royal Association for Disability and Rehabilitation)

12 City Forum
250 City Road
London EC1V 8AF
Tel: 020 7250 3222
Textphone: 020 7250 4119
Fax: 020 7250 0212
Website: www.radar.org.uk
Information about aids and mobility, holidays, sport and leisure for disabled people. Campaigns to improve the rights and care of disabled people. Sells special key to access locked disabled toilets.

REMAP

National Organiser
'Hazeldene'
Ightham
Sevenoaks
Kent TN15 9AD
Tel: 0845 1300 456
Fax: 0845 1300 789
Website: www.remap.org.uk
Makes or adapts aids, when not commercially available, for people with disabilities, at no charge to the disabled person. Has local branches.

Society of Teachers of the Alexander Technique (STAT)

1st floor, Linton House
39–51 Highgate Road
London NW5 1RS
Helpline: 0845 230 7828
Tel: 020 7284 3338
Fax: 020 7482 5435
Website: www.stat.org.uk
Offers general information and lists of teachers of the Alexander Technique in the UK and world-wide, and recommended training schools. Members receive up-to-date information.

Websites

A great deal of misinformation is out there on the internet. The following sites contain arthritis-related information that I find reliable.

www.altmedicine.com
Alternative Health News Online

www.altmednet.com
Alternative Medicine Alert

www.fda.gov/fdac
US Food and Drug Administration

www.nih.gov/niams
National Institute of Arthritis and Musculoskeletal and Skin Diseases (National Institutes of Health)

www.quackwatch.com
Quackery-related topics

Index

Have you found *Arthritis* useful and practical? If so, you may be interested in other books from Class Publishing.

Gout
the 'at your fingertips' guide £17.99
Professor Rodney Grahame,
Dr H Anne Simmonds
and Dr Elizabeth Carrey
This is an invaluable reference guide for people suffering from gout, which offers positive, practical advice on dealing with the condition, information on the causes of gout, and advice on the best ways to treat it and reduce chronic symptoms.

'It is excellent as an information resource for patients and doctors.'
Dr Michael L Snaith, University of Sheffield

Heart Health
the 'at your fingertips' guide £14.99
Dr Graham Jackson
This practical handbook, written by a leading cardiologist, answers all your questions about heart conditions. It tells you all about you and your heart, how to keep your heart healthy, or if it has been affected by heart disease – how to make it as strong as possible.

'Those readers who want to know more about the various treatments for heart disease will be much enlightened.'
Dr James Le Fanu, Daily Telegraph

Sexual Health for Men
the 'at your fingertips' guide £14.99
Dr Philip Kell and Vanessa Griffiths
This practical handbook answers hundreds of real questions from men with erectile dysfunction and their partners. Up to 50% of the population aged over 60 is impotent – though they need not be, if they take appropriate action.

'If you have any questions about sexual health and dysfunction, this is the book to answer them.' – Ann Tailor, Director, Sexual Dysfunction Association (formerly the Impotence Association)

Beating Depression
the 'at your fingertips' guide £17.99
Dr Stefan Cembrowicz
and Dr Dorcas Kingham
Depression is one of most common illnesses in the world – affecting up to one in four people at some time in their lives. *Beating Depression* shows sufferers and their families that they are not alone, and offers tried and tested techniques for overcoming depression.

'A sympathetic and understanding guide.'
Marjorie Wallace, Chief Executive, SANE

High Blood Pressure
the 'at your fingertips' guide £14.99
Dr Tom Fahey, Professor Deirdre Murphy
with Dr Julian Tudor Hart
The authors use all their years of experience as blood pressure experts to answer your questions on high blood pressure, in order to give you the information you need to bring your blood pressure down – and keep it down.

'Readable and comprehensive information' – Dr Sylvia McLaughlan, Director General, The Stroke Association

Dementia: Alzheimer's and other Dementias
the 'at your fingertips' guide £14.99
Harry Cayton, Dr Nori Graham
and Dr James Warner
At last – a book that tells you everything you need to know about Alzheimer's and other dementias. This book is an invaluable contribution to understanding all forms of dementia, and covers topics such as difficult behaviour, legal and financial implications of dementia and includes details of where to go for information and support.

'This book cannot be recommended too highly.' – Claire Rayner, Mail on Sunday

PRIORITY ORDER FORM

Cut out or photocopy this form and send it (post free in the UK) to:

Class Publishing Priority Service

FREEPOST

London W6 7BR

Please send me urgently
(tick boxes below)

*Post included
price per copy (UK only)*

☐ **Arthritis**
(ISBN 1 85959 106 X)   £17.99

☐ **Gout – the 'at your fingertips' guide**
(ISBN 1 85959 067 5)   £20.99

☐ **Heart Health – the 'at your fingertips' guide**
(ISBN 1 85959 097 7)   £17.99

☐ **Sexual Health for Men – the 'at your fingertips' guide**
(ISBN 1 85959 011 X)   £17.99

☐ **Beating Depression – the 'at your fingertips' guide**
(ISBN 1 85959 063 2)   £20.99

☐ **High Blood Pressure – the 'at your fingertips' guide**
(ISBN 1 85959 090 X)   £17.99

☐ **Dementia: Alzheimer's and other dementias – the
'at your fingertips' guide** (ISBN 1 85959 075 6)   £17.99

TOTAL _____

Easy ways to pay

Cheque: I enclose a cheque payable to Class Publishing for £ _____

Credit card: Please debit my ☐ Access ☐ Visa ☐ Amex

Number _____ Expiry date _____

Name _____

My address for delivery is _____

_____

Town _____ County _____ Postcode _____

Telephone number *(in case of query)* _____

Credit card billing address if different from above _____

_____

Town _____ County _____ Postcode _____

*Class Publishing's guarantee: remember that if, for any reason, you are not satisfied with these books, we will refund all
your money, without any questions asked. Prices and VAT rates may be altered for reasons beyond our control.*